Tapestry
of Health

Tapestry of Health

WEAVING WELLNESS INTO YOUR
LIFE THROUGH THE NEW SCIENCE OF
INTEGRATIVE MEDICINE

DANIEL A. MONTI, MD and
ANTHONY J. BAZZAN, MD

KALES
PRESS
in association with the
MARCUS INSTITUTE OF INTEGRATIVE HEALTH

Kenneth Kales, Editor and Publisher
Barbara J. Greenberg, Associate Editor
Susan Cane, Assistant Editor

Cover design by Laura Klynstra
Interior design by Jennifer Houle
Illustrations by Amy Saidens
Index by Schroeder Indexing Services

Library of Congress Cataloging-in-Publication Data

Names: Monti, Daniel A., author. | Bazzan, Anthony J., author.
Title: Tapestry of health : weaving wellness into your life through the new science of integrative medicine / Daniel A. Monti, MD, Anthony J. Bazzan, MD.
Description: San Diego : Kales Press, [2020] | Includes index. | Summary: "Preeminent leaders in the next generation of medicine present an essential guide to integrating multilayered healthcare approaches into one. Transforming the way you feel, think, look and thrive requires a healthcare approach that integrates all aspects of your well-being, including the physical, emotional, intellectual, spiritual, social and nutritional. Doctors Monti and Bazzan lay out, step-by-step, how to gain and maintain long-term vitality by integrating a broad range of restorative medicine, nutritional science, and healthy lifestyle practices. This convergence of time-honored approaches and cutting-edge technologies offers new preventions and cures while maintaining the fundamental principle that the parts cannot be well unless the whole is well. "This book is so incredibly timely and important because it helps you understand this new paradigm of health . . . You, as a patient, play the most important role in this shift as an active participant in behavioral, lifestyle, and dietary interventions so that these changes become woven into your daily life."—Sara Gottfried, MD, multiple New York Times bestselling author"—Provided by publisher.
Identifiers: LCCN 2019053333 (print) | LCCN 2019053334 (ebook) | ISBN 9780979845697 (hardcover) | ISBN 9781733395809 (ebook)
Subjects: LCSH: Integrative medicine.
Classification: LCC R733 .M66 2020 (print) | LCC R733 (ebook) | DDC 610—dc23
LC record available at https://lccn.loc.gov/2019053333
LC ebook record available at https://lccn.loc.gov/2019053334

Printed in the United States of America

First Edition

ISBN-13: 978-0-9798456-9-7 print edition
ISBN-13: 978-1-7333958-0-9 ebook edition

kalespress.com
San Diego, California

To our patients and their astounding human spirit

The part can never be well unless the whole is well

—PLATO

AUTHORS' NOTE

The medical conditions, diagnoses and treatment plans that we describe in individual patient stories are based on actual cases. The patients' names and backgrounds have been changed to protect their privacy. The information in this book is not intended or implied to be a diagnosis, treatment or substitution for consultation with your physician.

CONTENTS

FOREWORD

When I'm asked how I came to practice integrative and functional medicine, given that I was educated to be a mainstream physician, researcher and educator, my answer is surprisingly universal.

There are three key drivers. First, I witnessed another way—in my case, a great-grandmother who believed you don't find health in a pill bottle, you architect it with your daily life. Second, I was personally let down by conventional medicine. And third, there was an armful of revolutionary books that demonstrated a more effective way to create health.

This is one of those books.

As with the words and actions of my great-grandmother, when you read this book, you will grow to understand that an entire world of prevention, healing and repair exists through nutrition and lifestyle; that eating whole foods is the foundation of robust health; that you cannot survive without restorative sleep—the foundation upon which health begins—and that regular exercise and a contemplative practice can keep your body humming. All of this points to the need for a careful scientific examination, translated into an actionable plan, that is long overdue.

This book is the result of that kind of understanding, and will challenge you to think creatively and to question dogma. Even as I trained in the mainstream medical system, it occurred to me that something was terribly wrong. On one hand, US healthcare offers unparalleled innovation and scientific advances. On the other, the United States has the highest rate of obesity in the world, which leads to serious, costly and largely preventable diseases and conditions such as diabetes, high blood pressure, gallstones, stroke, sleep apnea, heart disease and cancer. Clearly, mainstream choices are not improving our health, especially when you consider that lifestyle choices are responsible for 70 percent of the cost of our nation's healthcare. If lifestyle is the chief cause of our rising healthcare costs, wouldn't lifestyle medicine make sense as our top priority?

Something else troubled me during my training: The disdain for nutrition and lifestyle approaches to chronic disease. I noted from the scientific literature that dietary and lifestyle approaches for diabetes worked better than medications, yet few physicians (myself included) were sufficiently educated in nutritional intervention or how to guide lifestyle changes. Among my brilliant professors at Harvard Medical School, none were interested in nutrition or lifestyle factors. They were Nobel Laureates who taught classes on genomics, immunology and translational aspects of molecular biology. When asked about lifestyle medicine, they would get pained looks on their faces and suggest perhaps I should consider the School of Public Health. I was confused, because the molecular influence of pharmaceuticals seemed similar to the molecular influence of food, exercise and sleep, yet somehow these approaches were considered less robust, even beneath the rigorous practice of medicine that was espoused in Boston.

Fortunately, the culture of medicine is changing. Medical doctors Daniel Monti and Anthony Bazzan are on the leading edge of changing this paradigm of medicine into something that encompasses true health, rather than simply managing disease. Both of them, like me, were trained in the conventional medical model and became disillusioned with our broken healthcare system. They are leaders in the field: compassionately treating patients, carefully educating the next generation of doctors and conducting rigorous research. They are intimately engaged in improved health in every facet imaginable. Their passion, caring and competence comes through in the book you are holding in your hands.

Dr. Monti completed his medical training at SUNY Buffalo School of Medicine and his residency at Thomas Jefferson University Hospital. He is a professor of psychiatry and emergency medicine at Thomas Jefferson University and their founding chair of the nation's first Integrative Medicine and Nutritional Sciences department at a medical school. Dr. Monti has authored dozens of medical journal articles, served as editor for medical textbooks, and is a coauthor of *Integrative Psychiatry and Brain Health*, which is part of the Andrew Weil Integrative Library. His research focuses on increasing quality of life and healing traumatic experiences for patients battling cancer, including through the application of mindfulness and the Neuro Emotional Technique, as described in this book so that anyone with a distressing history can unwind conditional responses. Additionally, Dr. Monti has performed landmark studies on nutritional interventions such as N-acetyl cysteine, a precursor of the master anti-oxidant glutathione, on clinical outcomes ranging from breast cancer to Parkinson's disease.

Dr. Bazzan was educated in Italy at the University of Padua School of Medicine and served his residency at Penn Presbyterian Medical Center. He completed fellowships at Albert Einstein Medical Center and Penn Presbyterian Medical Center. Dr. Bazzan is board-certified in internal medicine, a diplomate of the American Board of Integrative Holistic Medicine and a fellow of the American College of Nutrition. He is a disciple of Jeffery Bland, Ph.D., one of the founders of functional medicine. Dr. Bazzan's research focuses on nutritional and herbal treatments, hormone therapies and adjunctive care for mood disorders and cancer.

Both physicians are what we call in medicine the "triple threat"—that is, clinicians, researchers and educators. They mastered the art and science of modern medical care but also found it lacking, which is quite common among today's physicians. Sometimes doctors respond with withdrawal and burnout. Then there are the change agents, ignited to forge a new path forward. They don't dismiss one type of molecule over another or apply a reductionist approach. They are scientifically based. They understand the complexity of individual patients, their histories and narratives, and are genuinely curious about the manner in which their phenotype is expressed. They understand that there is an integrated whole that rests on the foundational complexity of network medicine.

This book is so valuable because it helps you find behaviors that may be slowly undermining your health and provides research-backed, realistic, easy-to-implement solutions to the problems that plague you, including stress, mood, fatigue and belly fat.

The future of medicine looks very different from what you've known until now. In the future, your doctor will better know you and your body and personally comprehend how your genetics are interacting with your environment, to eliminate much of the well-educated "guesswork" in clinical medicine. Doctors will be more comprehensive, communicative and connected to one another. Our lab work will pick up minor perturbations, and we will correct these with lifestyle and nutritional interventions before symptoms even appear. When serious illness occurs, we will understand our treatments and you, the patient, so well that we'll be able to prescribe lifestyle adjustments and treatments that are tailored just for you, including using medicines at personalized dosages to minimize or eliminate any side effects.

This book is so incredibly timely and important because it helps you understand this new paradigm of health—a massive shift that affects healthcare providers and patients alike. You, as a patient, play the most important role in this shift as an active participant in behavioral, lifestyle and dietary interventions so that these changes become woven into your daily life. Drs. Monti and Bazzan's cogent plan, based on proven dietary and lifestyle interventions integrated with modern medicine, is just what the doctor ordered. If you've picked up this book, you've already raised your hand and are now ready to take this path to true health!

SARA GOTTFRIED, MD
BERKELEY, CALIFORNIA

INTRODUCTION

Doctors Monti and Bazzan waste no time in *Tapestry of Health* to help you think, eat and live better. What strikes me most is their empathy all through their discussion. This book reveals physicians who care about you, care about helping you have the quality and enjoyment in life you deserve. At the same time, they help all of us think beyond traditional sick care to a vision of genuine health. I particularly love how their approach redefines the doctor-patient relationship as a proactive partnership with the singular goal of helping you to live your best life.

Without question, we need to bring health home. The twentieth century saw the ascendancy of the hospital, surrounded physically by diagnostic facilities, doctors' offices and medical schools. The results were revolutionary—new frontiers opened up to save lives in emergencies, to rescue those near death, to treat the worst diseases on the planet. Moreover, the individuals involved, the clinicians we treasure, continue to be dedicated, committed and inventive when helping a sick patient.

However, at the same time we achieved all this, the hospital model created a health care system that many see as sick. It is fragmented, forcing patients to navigate between specialists, diagnosticians, primary care providers and insurance companies. It is confusing, with precious little guidance to explain both costs and outcomes. And it is inequitable, with many people in the United States, and worldwide, unable to receive basic quality care.

When I look at the next revolution that will fix our system, I start with the person in the middle—you, the patient who will demand to be the pilot of her or his care. You, the individual who will want inalienable rights to health assurance, to getting and understanding an answer to the question, "What does this mean?" You, the person who will want to bring health home, to a place where your body and your home become the hub for living well. You, the person who will be guided to an understanding of how to prioritize thinking, eating, sleeping and loving.

For this revolution, I also look to clinical experts like Doctors Monti and Bazzan, both of whom know that medicine fails if it fails to address the whole person. We have spent too long separating mind and body, health and environment, relationships and well-being. For example, it sounds like a cliché to say that love is the best medicine—until you do the work that these authors have done to show how immensely powerful love is for our health.

The years that Doctors Monti and Bazzan have taught people how to weave a personal, dynamic and thriving health tapestry have generated the advocacy and support for integrative medicine by our friends at Thomas Jefferson University, including amazing philanthropists, a progressive board of trustees and a surrounding community that values what the integrative approach has to offer. And it is why we created the first in the nation Department of Integrative Medicine and Nutritional Sciences in a medical school, alongside a groundbreaking institute of integrative health that bears the name of the visionary who made it possible, philanthropist Bernard Marcus. The future will have plenty of robots to remember data—but really, our future depends on us appreciating human beings as wonderful, loving and healthy.

STEPHEN K. KLASKO, MD, MBA
PRESIDENT AND CEO, THOMAS JEFFERSON UNIVERSITY
AND JEFFERSON HEALTH

Tapestry
of Health

1

WEAVING A HEALTH TAPESTRY: RECLAIM YOUR BODY, MIND AND VITALITY

What is your plan for staying youthful and vibrant? How do you plan to improve your wellness—no matter how good or bad your current baseline is? How do you plan to stay in peak performance in your work, relationships, and mental, physical and emotional life? How do you plan to thrive more in the next ten years than you did in the last ten?

If you're still hoping to get these plans from your doctor, regrettably you'll likely be disappointed. That's because our current medical system isn't about keeping us vibrant, young, or at top performance levels. It's about putting out the fires of disease as quickly and economically as possible. That approach has its advantages in the short run, but it is only a small component of what we need "health" care to be. As a nation, Americans rank abysmally low for healthy life expectancy, and our overall performance as we age is being increasingly dragged down by health burdens that are entirely avoidable. There is not nearly enough preventive medicine, and a separate model for recovery medicine from an illness is sorely needed. Enter the new field of *integrative* medicine.

The US arguably has the best *conventional* medicine in the world. Our technology outshines everyone else's, our surgical techniques have revolutionized the operating room, our vaccines have eradicated terrible diseases, our training attracts health professionals from all over the world, and our research and scholarly pub-lications far surpass those of any other country. Why then is our population so unwell? Why do we keep losing performance points, and even IQ points? Clearly more medicine does not equal more health.

The answers are complex, in part because health care is complex. But it's also because of a lack of imagination. Medicine has largely boxed itself in with a dis-ease-based model, where the focus is on putting out fires—an infection that needs an antibiotic or a troubled organ that needs surgery. To continue with this fire analogy, the conventional approach does little to clear away brush and safeguard flammables to maintain a healthy and safe perimeter around your home and thus minimize the risk of damage. Home is your body and mind, and the healthy perimeter is your immune system. In fact, the insurance companies have "ensured" that your health care providers spend as little face time with you as possible by building in a reward system that favors the quantity of patients they see over the quality of care they pro-vide. In that system, health care is mostly constrained by pharmaceutical, surgical and therapeutic algorithms that are based on short-term outcomes of a disease state such as a drug to lower cholesterol versus long-term cardiovascular wellness.

The insurance companies' demands lead to constraints on physicians' time, along with physicians' inadequate training on wellness interventions, compound the problem. For example, a recent article in the *Journal of the American Medical Association* underscored the inadequate training doctors receive on diet and nutri-tion. While most currently practicing doctors understand that diet is an import-ant factor in wellness, they don't have strong enough training about this correlation and have little encouragement to pursue it. Then there's what would seem to be the obvious, yet is hiding in plain sight—living with vitality takes more than just being free of disease.

In the earliest civilizations, people sought healing through some mixture of will and mysticism, combined with natural resources such as medicinal plants and hot springs. Clearly they had a lot of limitations in curing health problems. Although humanity has moved on to where we now benefit from huge advances in modern medicine, it's important to remind ourselves that some of those healing gems from thousands of years ago are still valuable today.

As one example, many great cures have come from the plant world. In fact, the oldest written evidence of a healing plant preparation dates back about 5,000 years ago to ancient India. Their "pharmacy" at the time included approximately 250 plants, some of which are still known today, such as the poppy, while others such as mandrake have fallen away with the passage of time. Ancient Chinese writings from around 2,500 BC reveal the use of many botanicals that are still easily found in grocery stores today, such as ginseng and cinnamon. About 40 percent of prescription medicines come from plant extracts or synthesized plant compounds, but beyond these we do not recommend many unregulated botanical preparations because of potential drug interactions. We do, however, advocate a plant-based diet and eating as many edible plants in their natural state as possible. The potential benefits to health and wellness in the phytonutrients they contain are enormous. Also, some of the rituals and meditative practices of yesterday are tremendously relevant today in proven wellness programs like Mindfulness-Based Stress Reduction (MBSR).

Our integrative approach to health and wellness, in close collaboration with the Marcus Foundation and the leadership of Thomas Jefferson University in Philadelphia, led our team to create the Marcus Institute of Integrative Health. Building on that foundation, in 2019 we created the first department of Integrative Medicine and Nutritional Sciences at a conventional medical school in the country, perhaps the world. Jefferson takes a leading role in the Integrative Health revolution by putting this new department on par with medicine, surgery, anesthesiology, neurology, pediatrics and all of the other medical departments that comprise a medical college. This historic first reflects that the medical establishment is beginning to recognize something additional is needed for the overall picture of good health. Integrating the tremendous medical science that exists with cutting-edge technologies and wellness strategies is what our department and institute is about, and what this book is about.

Our clinical programs include lessons from history combined with the most advanced technology available today. In our view it isn't an either/or situation of going natural or going strictly modern medicine—there are pluses and minuses to both approaches. But by combining the two and integrating the value from each, we have found that our patients not only heal faster from their conditions, they remain healthier longer through a fundamental understanding that wellness builds synergistically from a healthy lifestyle and focused medical care.

It's important here to distinguish between popping a pill and changing the way you live in order to achieve your optimum level of health. Popping a pill may cure a disease state, or may lead to a long-term dependency on those pharmaceuticals, but at best it's a one-dimensional approach. To transform your level of wellness so that you can think better, feel better and perform better is a multi-dimensional endeavor, operating in a results-oriented integrative medicine model that opens a world of solutions and options you might not have known were even there.

Our goal is to challenge you to redefine what's possible for your health and happiness, to share with you what we have learned and witnessed, and to give you the tools to take your quality of life to the next level. Some of the most common statements we hear from our patients are, "Why didn't anyone tell me about this when I was thirty?" Or forty-five, or sixty. The answer is the medical community hasn't been convinced of this, and it's only fairly recently that there have been enough of us to get their attention. Our patients remind us of this struggle every day with stories of needless dysfunction and suffering as a result of the integrative medicine we practice not having been available to them before.

Each new discovery in applying additional options to patient care opens our minds to new possibilities for the prevention of disease and long-lasting wellness. For example, the leading edge of research on brain plasticity shows that brain cells can regenerate and neurotransmitters can recharge. Every day millions of Americans apply this discovery for improving their mental functioning without most of them even knowing it—from those doing crossword puzzles to those doing ten-second mindfulness techniques. We also know that other aspects of physiology affect the brain and vice versa; for example the gut-brain connection—every day millions of Americans apply this by deciding to quit sugary beverages and increase their use of natural teas to improve gut-brain health, just one of so many exciting wellness options. You are among the pioneers in an emerging movement that first considers each person's uniqueness, and then empowers each to take personalized health-promoting, vitality-enhancing steps.

The metaphor of a tapestry's elegant art form applies well here. Like your own well-being, a tapestry requires time, caring and purposefulness in taking into account the threads, stitches, patterns and colors—none of which on their own would achieve the extraordinary creation possible by weaving together all of these elements.

As practitioners of Integrative and Nutritional Medicine, we don't claim to have all of the answers; not by any means. The two of us are evolving as physicians just as the field of medicine is. However, what we can say with confidence is: an integrated approach that shares the responsibility of modern traditional approaches as well as the wisdom of some nontraditional ones with patients as active partners is the new wave in health care. We encourage your intuition so that you listen to your body, mind and spirit, and learn some proven strategies to weaving together a healthier, happier and more vibrant life.

2

WEAVING IN OPTIMAL NUTRITION

Food is at the foundation of our integrative approach. The right nutrition is crucial to you feeling your best, thinking your best, performing your best and looking your best. What we eat can feed and nourish the cells of the body, or pollute them and create diseases. Some foods are what we call "givers"; that is, they give us energy and sustenance, while others are what we refer to as "takers" because they have a toxic and draining effect. We are a resilient species and can tolerate some takers, but the problem with the typical American or "Western" diet is that it is made up of almost all takers. No wonder chronic health issues are so pervasive in the US. In this section we will teach you how to maximize the givers and avoid the takers. Quite simply, the right foods can help keep you be trim, hormonally balanced, metabolically tuned, emotionally centered and more.

To look better, feel better and perform better, eat better. Eat better? What does that really mean? Rather than focusing on calories and the scale, focus more on the givers. For example, when you eat raw vegetables and fruits, a percentage of the sunlight's photons involved in their growth process, known as photosynthesis, remains in their cells and gets transferred to you. We call it "eating sunlight" or "eating living food."

On the opposite side are the takers. We call eating those "eating dead food." They include all red meat, all luncheon meats, all dairy including cheese and yogurt, all refined flour and sugar, and all foods that are canned, preserved, fortified, genetically modified or deep fried. This goes for some brands of so-called healthier vegan alternatives like fake hotdogs, burgers, bacon, cheeses, chicken—the list is getting longer every day—that may save you from some of the perils of eating their animal counterparts, but these products are usually highly processed with large amounts of sodium, preservatives and other chemicals. There are exceptions, which is why we teach our patients to read labels carefully. Takers are linked to high risks for inflammatory autoimmune diseases, heart disease and depression among other conditions. Plus they are linked to addiction to sugar, sodium and other flavor enhancers that lead to obesity while actually being under-nourishing, which helps explain why a lot of Americans are overfed but undernourished.

Inflammatory foods are now considered to be among the most dangerous factors in both long-term diseases such as heart disease, cancer, diabetes and asthma, as well as in short-term illnesses such as colds, headaches, acid reflux and allergies. The Western diet is an inflammatory nightmare. Here's a little etymology: inflammation comes from the Latin verb *inflammare* (to inflame). For thousand of years the five cardinal signs of inflammation have been redness, heat, pain, swelling and loss of function. When we are inflamed we are literally burning, like meat on a barbecue. This means all of the "-itises" you hear about, like arthritis or colitis, point to burning of that body part: arthritis means the joints are on fire, colitis the colon is on fire, and so on. Takers fuel fires, givers put them out.

Our Health Tapestry Meal Plan is full of performance givers. We believe that eating the way we prescribe also helps you maintain balanced PH levels in your body tissues and fluids; slightly more alkaline than acidic. This tilt toward alkalinity decreases inflammation. Alkaline friendly foods are mainly vegetables, especially green leafy ones, some whole grains, and some fruits. Also included are plenty of anti-inflammatory plant-based fats like avocados and almonds, versus pro-inflammatory fats from meat and dairy.

There's another link between food and inflammation and it's shaking up the world. In the past two years, scientific studies have revealed the presence in the body of superfamilies of anti-inflammatory molecules known as Specialized Pro-Resolving Mediators (SPMs)—they are derivatives of omega-3s, the healthy fats you hear so much about that are prevalent in many fish such as wild salmon and some plant sources like flax seeds.

Here's the really good news: they are naturally occurring molecules that increase with good nutrition, exercise, sleep and an overall healthy lifestyle. When our patients need additional anti-inflammatory support beyond diet and other lifestyle interventions, we recommend specific supplemental nutrients. Throughout the book we include web addresses for supplements we recommend so you can check them out. Most of the products we recommend in our practice are available on the Marcus Institute website (https://marcusstore.jeffersonhealth.org /collections/shop). With few exceptions, we do not directly financially benefit if you choose to order a product. Proceeds go to the Marcus Institute, which is a component of the university. The overwhelming benefit to us is that we have these nutritional tools readily available for the patients we serve.

Having these nutrient-based tools allows us to give patients the needed support to address inflammation with less likelihood of creating bad side effects like those common from the use of anti-inflammatory drugs. A whole new narrative on healthcare has taken flight since the discovery of the effects of inflammation and natural ways to reduce it. One outbranch is a new theory that the chronic inflammatory conditions common in older age are a result of the body's lower generation of SPMs, similarly to how other bodily systems slow down with aging. Many years before this discovery, we had developed our plant-based Health Tapestry Meal Plan that continues to be supported by the latest published research in the field.

"Hold on a minute," you might be saying now. "If I don't eat lots of meat, how will I get enough protein?" Good question, and it's one that comes up a lot from our patients. The conversation goes something like this. Let's call the patient Henry:

"Doc, I know you mean well but do I look like the kind of person who can live on rabbit food?"

"I understand what you're saying. And yes, this is a different way of thinking. So let me ask you something. Have you ever seen an elephant?"

"Of course I have."

"Do you think there's enough meat on an elephant?"

"Yeah, they're huge."

"About six or seven tons."

"That big? Wow." Henry nods his head.

"Yeah. Do you know what they eat?"

"Uh . . . hay? I mean at the zoo they feed them hay and peanuts I guess."

"That's right. And in the wild they feed on grass, leaves, bushes, twigs and roots. They're complete vegans. No meat, no fish, just whatever plants they find."

"So I'm guessing you're going to tell me to give up my filet mignon."

"Well, Henry—"

"And hamburger? What if it's lean? Don't even answer. I already know what you're going to say: 'Only in moderation.'"

"Sure. You can do fish, too. Or chicken and turkey, in moderation as you said."

"All right, Doc. So I know this is going to sound crazy but how does an elephant end up as an elephant if all it eats are plants? How does it get enough protein?"

That's when we pull the curtain back and reveal the protein myth. Proteins are chains of amino acids strung together like pearls in a necklace. There are about twenty amino acids on our planet and they are most commonly found in humans and other animals. If there is a total of twenty amino acids in each of the estimated 20,000 to 25,000 human gene proteins, how many possible amino acid sequences are there? A gazillion. Let's leave the math to your liver as it converts the food you eat into the building blocks of amino acids and proteins you need. The point is, there are lots of ways to get enough protein from plants such as beans, nuts, soy and some whole grains, as well as minimally processed protein extracts from peas, hemp and other plant sources.

To simplify, you use your teeth, tongue, saliva, gastric juices, pancreatic juices, and more to break down food into single amino acids, fats and carbohydrates that are absorbed by your gut and sent to your liver. The liver then uses those building blocks to build your body. The healthier the food, the healthier the body. Unprocessed plant protein sources are all on the upside. While many animal protein sources are on the downside, particularly with their saturated fats that contribute to digestive, cardiovascular and inflammatory disorders and weight gain, to name a few. Our overall recommendation of 60 to 90 grams of protein a day for adults remains the same, whether from plant-based sources or in moderate combination with animal-based ones. If you are highly active then you may need more protein.

So much for the protein myth. But there are other meat-related myths lined up to take its place. Ones propped up by popular advertising slogans like "Beef. It's what's for dinner" and "Pork. The Other White Meat." Let's do some more myth busting.

Overwhelmingly consistent findings in wide-ranging scientific studies show just how destructive eating more than moderate amounts of meat is to our health. Research links the consumption of fat-saturated meats and dairy products with increased rates of heart disease, stroke, high blood pressure, high cholesterol, diabetes and many cancers including breast, prostate and colon cancer. The story is even worse for processed meats like pepperoni and most deli meats used in sandwiches. In fact, the World Health Organization (WHO) has issued alerts that processed meats, defined as any that have been altered from their natural state "through salting, curing, fermentation, smoking, or other processes to enhance flavor or improve preservation" are "carcinogenic." These include some of the most popular items at your neighborhood store: deli slices, smoked ham, hot dogs, bacon, sausage, beef jerky, and more.

There is a lot of research showing that many men eat meat because they think it is a good way to boost their testosterone levels. You can do your own quick research on this just by going online and googling "ways to increase male testosterone" and you'll see more than enough cheerleading to eat saturated-fat meat to build muscle and increase sexual performance. That's another myth. While sufficient protein and other nutrients are needed for adequate testosterone production, it has been shown that a diet too high in protein can actually *lower* testosterone levels. We suspect this is particularly the case for animal protein, not to mention its higher risk for heart disease, diabetes and enlarged prostate, among other illnesses.

But here's the real irony in their drive for masculinity. Over time, this kind of diet can actually *reduce* a man's sexual proclivities. Sluggishness sets in, blood circulation slows, belly fat accumulates, self-esteem suffers. A healthier approach to raising testosterone levels is to eat legumes, green leafy vegetables, chia seeds and avocados among other plant-based sources, without any risks. We will get into the details as you read on.

Another myth is that "fat" is bad for you. But there is bad and good fat. Bad fat is bad for you and good fat is good for you. It is just as important to go out of your way to eat good fat as it is to go out of your way to avoid bad fat.

We rank fats as worst, bad, better and best. The worst fats are the saturated kinds that you mostly find in meat and dairy, as well as a few plant sources such as palm. Thankfully, the door has been closed on the separate monstrously bad saturated fat called trans fat—effective June 18, 2018, the Food and Drug Administration banned the use of man-made trans fats, also referred to as partially hydrogenated oils, thus requiring food manufacturers to rid this health hazard from our food chain. This is a real triumph for public health. It needs to be noted that there are naturally occurring trans fats in some foods; however these are at low levels and considered to be safe. We recommend no more than five percent of your caloric intake each day contain saturated fat. Thus, a standard 2,000 calories per day would mean 10 grams or less of saturated fats.

We categorize omega-6 fats as bad fats for most Americans. While it is essential to get some of them, the typical Western diet has a tremendous excess of them. The problem is that the foods high in omega-6 fat are pro-inflammatory. These include peanuts and oils from corn and soybeans.

FOOD HIGH IN WORST FATS

FOOD	GRAMS OF BAD FAT
Light Whipping Cream	23 in 1 cup
Rich Chocolate Ice Cream	15 in 1 cup
Braised Beef Short Ribs	15 in 3 oz
Chocolate Creme Pie	15 in 1 serving
Roast Pork Ribs	15 in 1 rack
Ricotta Cheese	10 in 1/2 cup
Prime Rib Steak	9 in 3 oz
Whole Milk	9 in 16 oz glass

Conversely, good fats are unsaturated and often referred to as monosaturates and polyunsaturates. Omega-9 fats fit in this category. Foods high in them include avocados, olives, extra-virgin olive oil and some nuts. We note that plant foods and animal foods generally have a mix of fat types even if there is a preponderance of one over the others. The best fats are omega-3's, found mostly in several types of fresh food such as wild salmon, flax seeds and chia seeds. Foods high in omega-3 and omega-9 fats are anti-inflammatory. The goal is to keep the omega-3 to omega-6 ratio as high as possible. The more omega-3 (and probably omega-9) fats we consume, the better we can counter the inflammation causing effects of excessive omega-6's and other inflammatory foods.

FOOD HIGH IN GOOD FATS

FOOD	GRAMS OF GOOD FAT IN 3.5 OZ SERVING
Olive Oil	80
Safflower Oil	75
Brazil Nuts	48
Almonds	43
Flax Seeds	27
Pumpkin Seeds	25
Avocado	15
Salmon	11

Research suggests that proactively increasing good fat consumption may serve as preventive healthcare, possibly by shutting down inflammation before it has a chance to even get started. A large study published in the *New England Journal of Medicine* showed that a diet rich in omega-3s and omega-9s had notably superior cardiovascular outcomes than a so-called fat free diet.

Interestingly, meat has both types of fat—good and bad—but the omega-3 to omega-6 ratio has gotten much worse over the past few decades. This is likely due to livestock being raised quite differently than it was 50 years ago. The meadow grass that cows used to eat has largely been replaced by corn byproducts, and gruel is known to be the cause of serious livestock diseases. This is why some claim that livestock that is truly free range or in the case of beef, grass fed, is healthier. That is potentially true; however, we still suggest eating as little meat as possible, especially in midlife, and beyond then it's best that it be as lean as possible. Fresh fish and vegan sources of protein are recommended as a replacement whenever possible.

Now on to the next myth:

"Got Milk?"

We sure hope not. But the commercials are funny.

"Milk Does a Body Good."

Not so fast. That's not what the research says.

"Milk Builds Strong Bones."

Does it though? One compelling study showed worse bone health in terms of fracture risk with higher dairy consumption. While it's still being debated whether milk is good for infants, there's enough evidence for us to conclude that drinking milk beyond infancy is not healthy. The protein casein is an allergen for some and possibly carcinogenic in large quantities, the fat is like eating the end of a pork chop, and the sugar—lactose—becomes indigestible as we age, creating what is referred to as lactose intolerance. Worldwide, about 65 percent of the adult population is lactose intolerant. As many as 95 percent of East Asians, 75 percent of African and Caribbean people, and 50 percent of Mediterranean people are lactose intolerant. The conventional wisdom has been that drinking milk into adulthood is normal and to not be able to do so—because of lactose intolerance—is a disorder. But many researchers are breaking away: it isn't normal at all and the disorder is not in stopping, but in continuing to consume milk. Though there are those who are lactose tolerant and can continue to digest milk without apparent issues into their adulthood, we still advise minimizing consumption of all dairy products including cheese, butter, cream and yogurt due to their fat content and inflammatory effects.

We anticipate you will see the advantages of our Health Tapestry Meal Plan. We urge you to try it strictly for at least three weeks. At the end of that trial period, we believe you'll begin to see a transformation in how you look and feel—lighter, healthier and more energetic. We hope you will be so thrilled with the results that you too will stay on the eating plan forever as a part of your revitalized lifestyle, as so many of our patients have.

Cooked plants are fine, but raw ones are better; eat both. While white potatoes should be avoided completely, some other root vegetables can be included in smaller amounts (one serving per day), particularly orange, yellow and red vegetables such as carrots, beets, squash, red and yellow peppers and yams. As you read on, you will see several tasty snack options and some terrific recipes and meal plans.

GETTING STARTED

Practice Mindful Eating: Think about everything you put in your body and ask yourself if it's a giver or a taker. Do not eat while watching television or doing other things. Eat in a relaxed environment and be sure to chew each mouthful five to 10 times.

Drink Five to Eight Glasses of Water a Day: If you are hydrated, you will be less hungry and more healthy.

Eat Breakfast Everyday: It is critical to eat breakfast, but in a different way than you are used to. Morning is a great time to have some vegetable protein, such as one of the shakes we recommend (see below) or to use your rice cooker or steamer to prepare a variety of fresh grains and/or greens.

Eat Plenty of Veggies for Lunch and Dinner: Vegetables should be the main food group at lunch and dinner. Fill three-quarters of your plate with veggies, and any variety of protein sources and whole grains can make up the remainder.

Listen to Your Gut: If a food makes you feel bad, it is probably bad for you! Take note of how certain foods make you feel after you eat them.

Enjoy One or Two Healthy Snacks a Day at Work or School: Raw vegetables, raw walnuts and vegan yogurt are three great examples (more below).

Eat Fresh Fruits: Generally speaking, the Health Tapestry Meal Plan allows for one to two servings of dark, fleshy fruit per day. Good fruits include plums and berries, which are rich in phytonutrients. Avoid commercial bananas and most grapes because they have high glycemic indexes, and dried fruits because they contain a lot of sugar and often are laced with unwanted chemical preservatives. If you are trying to lose weight limit yourself to a high fiber fruit such as an apple, which helps fill you up.

Eat Fresh Sprouts: Add sprouts to your salads and sandwiches and/or drink up to two ounces of wheat grass juice daily.

Blend Veggie Smoothies: Smoothies are a great way to get your greens in every day. To make it easy, we suggest using one of our meal replacement shakes as a base and then adding other healthy ingredients like a handful of spinach.

Eat Only Whole, Unprocessed Grains: Avoid refined, polished and processed foods such as pasta, rice, bread, crackers and chips. Grains in general are best eaten in moderation. Focus on vegetables.

Avoid Fried Foods: Deep fried foods are high in calories and bad fats.

Avoid Processed Commercial Deli Meats: The best form of animal protein is fresh, wild fish (up to three servings per week); fish has the added bonus of healthy omega fat. Beef, pork, lamb and other red meats are best to avoid, though small amounts of lean grass-fed beef are okay for some, as are moderate amounts of lean poultry white meat.

If You Do Eat Animal Protein, Do So with Green Veggies Only: It is crucial not to mix animal proteins with grains and simple carbs for optimal digestion. Add some extra-virgin olive oil to the meal so that its polyphenols and anti-inflammatory properties can help balance against consuming unhealthy animal fat.

Choose Condiments Low in Sugar and Salt: Try Bragg Liquid Aminos in place of soy sauce, salsa in place of ketchup, and pesto and vegan mayo.

One of the beautiful things about our program is its built-in flexibility. For instance, if you don't like a particular food, don't eat it—neither of us would touch turnips no matter how rich they are in vitamins A, C, E, and B-complex, omegas, protein and minerals. You likely have your own "never gonna do it" foods. That's okay. There are plenty of other choices. A fundamental part of this all is to enjoy yourself within the general framework and not be a slave to your diet. Here are a few more basic guidelines:

Eat Three Meals and Two Snacks a Day. Breakfast, lunch and dinner, along with one snack in the late morning and one in the late afternoon. However, don't starve yourself or overeat. For women, we recommend 1,500 to 2,000 calories per day and for men 2,000 to 2,500. If you are trying to lose weight start with the low end of the guideline and take off another 250 calories if needed, and vice versa if you are trying to gain weight—add 250.

Eat Enough Food. The foods we recommend like leafy greens are nutrient dense and low calorie. You have to eat a lot of them to be full. As you transition to this diet, aim to eat about three to four pounds of food, but the right food, every day. You will have a hard time being successful if you don't eat enough pounds of food, otherwise your body will send hunger signals to your brain. Most people feel very satisfied at about four pounds of food. The number one mistake dieters make is to not eat enough—they feel starved and then shovel down food to compensate. If you keep track of your food consumption in aggregate pounds, satiety will result. The trick is what the pounds are made of, and that's where our food guide comes in. For example, four pounds of raw veggies is about 400 calories; four pounds of sugary breakfast cereal is about 10,000 calories. But the volume of veggies to get you to four pounds is several times that of processed, dense foods like luncheon meat, French fries, cheese, etc.

Divide Your Plate into Four Quarters. Fill three-quarters of your lunch and dinner plates with vegetables and the remaining quarter with your choice of proteins or whole grains, not both. Note: If you stray, at least avoid animal protein and grains at the same meal because that combination is hard on your digestive system. When you are done, refill your plate with another salad or veggies of some sort. Be mindful of getting enough pounds of food, as described above.

Drink Filtered Water or Herbal or Green Tea. Avoid soda, caffeinated beverages, alcohol, fruit juices and dairy milk. We also recommend unsweetened nondairy milk such as almond, soy, flax and rice.

If Trying to Lose Weight, Eat Fruit Only a Couple of Days Each Week but Limit to One Serving Each of Those Days. Fruit contains fructose, a natural sugar that can raise your glycemic levels just like other sugars do. Avoid fruit juices and dried fruit because they contain even more concentrated sugars. High fiber fruit like an organic apple as a snack when you're hungry can be a good option, especially if you are trying to lose weight.

Filling three-quarters of your plate with vegetables at every lunch and dinner meal equals at least seven servings a day. One serving equals half a cup of cooked vegetables, but the truth is you can eat an unlimited amount of most vegetables. Highlights include green leafy vegetables such as spinach, romaine lettuce, kale, collards and chard, and cruciferous vegetables such as red cabbage, cauliflower, broccoli and Brussels sprouts. Exceptions to keep in mind are potatoes, corn, carrots and other vegetables high in carbohydrates because those more readily convert to sugar.

Juicing is popular, and we often are asked about its benefits. Theoretically you can drink a concentration of absorbable nutrients in one glass that otherwise might take you all day to chew those same vegetables and fruits. However, because juicing removes some nutrients, and most importantly the pulp, we prefer making smoothies so as not to lose the pulp and its wonderful healthful properties. Nonetheless some folks love to juice and we encourage it if that's your preference. One note, though: it is important to balance juiced carrots or apples with greens such as kale, collards, spinach, celery and bell peppers. We generally do not recommend carrot juice on its own because of the high amount of natural sugar, and suggest that you only include in your juice blend one to two carrots or one fruit (e.g., an apple or handful of berries) at most each day.

We also recommend "eating the rainbow," meaning go colorful with your vegetable choices, from the common orange yam, yellow bell pepper, red tomato, purple potato, green beans and white cauliflower to the exotic orange Cinderella pumpkin, yellow delicata squash, red bitter radicchio, purple Sicilian eggplant, green lacinato kale and white napa cabbage.

Going with organic vegetables and fruits and limiting eggs and meat as much as possible is a good idea. Mounting evidence shows that pesticides, pollutants and genetically modified organisms (GMOs) can compromise the human immune system and thus lead to more illness. Your immune system is built to fight off most invaders, but what concerns us is the cumulative toll toxins take on our bodies day after day, year after year.

Think about this analogy using a river. If you put some pollutants in a river, the water will cleanse itself through a natural downstream flow. But if you keep putting in more and more pollutants every day of every year, then the river won't be able to keep up and eventually will become dirty. If you stopped the dumping and proactively worked toward restoration, over time the river would return to its natural state. Real world examples of this ecological restoration from polluted to clean include Massachusetts's Charles River, Ohio's Ashtabula River and Virginia's James River—all three ecosystems are flourishing again.

Your body is similar. You are already dealing with a lot you don't have much control over, such as car exhaust, medications and urban life stress. But you do have a lot of control over what you eat and whether or not you want to include pesticide and fertilizer residue in your diet. Admittedly, there is controversy as to whether organically grown food has higher nutritional value. What is indisputable though is that it is cleaner. A 2014 publication in the *British Journal of Nutrition* found that organically grown crops were less likely to contain detectable levels of pesticides, and because of differences in fertilization techniques, they were also nearly half as likely to test positive for certain toxic heavy metals.

There are other practical considerations in thinking about switching to organic—a main one being the cost to you as a consumer. On average, organic produce is about 30 percent more expensive than conventionally grown produce. That extra amount can really add up and be unaffordable for many. If you are among these many, no need to worry: conventionally grown produce still has lots of nutrients to offer, including self-generating antioxidants that can help fight against pesticide and fertilizer residues.

If you can stretch your budget a bit, you can buy some organic produce along with some conventionally grown. Think of it as selective purchasing. With that said, some vegetables and fruits are priorities because they have heavier amounts of toxic residues. Those have been nicknamed "The Dirty Dozen" by the Environmental Working Group (EWG) and it is highly recommended that they be purchased in organic varieties. Even if you thoroughly wash and peel these conventionally grown twelve, tests reveal a frightening picture. It's not just the outside skin to be concerned with; those pesticides and fertilizers are absorbed and integrated into the plant fibers. The most recent list of "The Dirty Dozen" starting with the worst follows:

1. Strawberries
2. Apples
3. Nectarines
4. Peaches
5. Celery
6. Grapes
7. Cherries
8. Spinach
9. Tomatoes
10. Sweet bell peppers
11. Cherry tomatoes
12. Cucumbers

On the other side of the equation are what the EWG calls "The Clean 15." These foods contain relatively low amounts of pesticide or fertilizer residue. The most recent list of "The Clean 15" starting with the best follows:

1. Avocados
2. Sweet corn
3. Pineapples
4. Cabbage
5. Frozen sweet peas
6. Onions
7. Asparagus
8. Mangoes
9. Papayas
10. Kiwis
11. Eggplant
12. Honeydew melon
13. Grapefruit
14. Cantaloupe
15. Cauliflower

These lists can help you with your grocery shopping. For instance, if you want cucumbers it is better to get the organic ones and if you want avocados it is okay to get the conventional ones.

Now that we have covered the plan for three-quarters of your plate to be vegetables, and to refill that part of your plate especially if they are raw veggies, let's talk about the remaining quarter for proteins or grains.

First, proteins. We recommend a combination of large amounts of plant-based ones and small amounts of animal-based ones. Good sources for plant-based protein include beans, nuts, peas, hemp and whole grains. Soy (non-GMO) is also good; however we recommend limiting your consumption to only one serving a day equaling a maximum of one cup of soy milk, tofu, tempeh, or other soy-based foods. This restriction is also partly due to unresolved research about how the naturally occurring isoflavones found in soy affect estrogen levels.

For moderate amounts of animal-based protein, we recommend only two sources. The first is a select group of fish: those that are omega-3 rich catches such as salmon, albacore tuna, bluefish, herring and Atlantic mackerel, and low-fat, white-fleshed, cold-water, deep-ocean varieties such as cod, haddock and sole. Please keep in mind two basic guidelines for buying fish: 1) Buy domestically harvested catches, not imported varieties, as American waters are reliably cleaner than most overseas fishing grounds; and 2) buy wild varieties rather than farm-raised ones. Wild fish have a higher nutritional value and taste better. The only other animal protein source we recommend is egg white from chicken eggs that are grown free range without hormones, pesticides or antibiotics. If you still want poultry, chicken or turkey that is grown free range without hormones, pesticides or antibiotics is the best option.

Now on to grains. Let's start with the elephant in the room—gluten. There is compelling evidence showing the downside to grains containing gluten. But a common misperception about grains is similar to the one we discussed earlier about fats. There are good fats and bad fats. There are also good grains and bad grains. The fact is, gluten-free, whole, unprocessed grains are good for you and do not cause problems for most people. They are rich in the vitamin B family, protein, antioxidants, trace minerals, fiber and more. Healthy gluten-free grains include brown rice, wild rice, buckwheat (despite its name, there is no wheat in buckwheat), millet, oats, quinoa and amaranth.

3

HEALTH TAPESTRY MEAL PLAN

What follows is a blueprint for making some Health Tapestry Meal Plan dishes. Feel free to add your own twists as our plan is meant to be flexible within reason. It may seem like a lot to think about at first, but with a little practice you will understand the basics well enough to have them memorized.

Since you don't have to worry about portion sizes when it comes to most fresh vegetables, especially the leafy greens and cruciferous ones, it's okay to pile your plate high—when you have a big appetite you might need more than twice the volume of vegetables to equal the calories of processed foods. Besides, your body has built-in mechanisms to signal when you've had your fill of fresh vegetables; a signal that gets muted when you eat processed foods.

RETHINK BREAKFAST

To start your day off right, the first step is to realize healthy breakfast food is not what it used to be. Today, according to the most recent research, less than 20 percent of Americans regularly have a traditional breakfast, and this number is projected to drop. Instead, for those who do eat breakfast, they have turned to snack bars, bagels, yogurt, and as you might imagine, increasingly to fast-food breakfast sandwiches that are filled with unhealthy processed meats, processed cheese, a ton of sodium and all kinds of chemical additives. The fact is fewer Americans are eating any breakfast. Only about one-third of us have breakfast, meaning two-thirds go without it altogether. Yet it is important to not only start the day off with food, but with *healthy* food. If you don't like having a full breakfast, or prefer something light to start off with and then have a midmorning snack, that is fine. Eating something will help you to make better choices for lunch and dinner.

One way out of this downward trend is to look to other countries for inspiration. For instance, in Japan white rice and miso soup, in India vegetable stew with steamed lentils, and in Costa Rica black beans and mango are popular breakfasts.

So why not try combining several whole grains such as oat groats, quinoa, brown rice and amaranth in your rice cooker when you first wake up? In about the same time it will take you to shower and get dressed, your grains will be ready. Then mix in a few almonds or seeds, a sprinkling of your favorite herbs and some soy/almond/rice/flax milk, or just enjoy as is. If you eat grains for breakfast, consider that to be your grain intake for the whole day and do not have them with your other meals.

A plant-based protein shake derived from hemp or peas is also a great and easy breakfast. There are many products available commercially. Choose whichever ones work best for you. We often recommend Pro-Meal Advanced powder for those looking for a shake that helps to maximize fitness. These supplements mix very easily in a blender, or even in a convenient blender bottle with some cold water and then shaken. They are great substitutes for whichever meal of the day you want help with—that's breakfast for a lot of folks.

You can also use the shake as a smoothie base. Just add a handful of greens and blend for a super power-packed meal. Other healthy add-ins include flax seeds, almond butter and fresh berries. Other foods to bring in more plant-based protein to your morning include avocado toast, sautéed vegetables and a tofu scramble.

AT CENTER STAGE: LUNCH AND DINNER

Lunch and dinner offer many creative options for the three-quarters of your plate being vegetables guideline to really take hold. Change is often difficult, so this shift may take a little getting used to. If you need to build up to this ratio over a few day or weeks, that is fine. Vegetable soups and vegetable-based smoothies and juices also count toward your three-quarters goal.

At least four times a week include cruciferous vegetables in your meals—they are among the crown jewels of vegetables in that they offer concentrations of special phytonutrients. The most common of the crucifers are broccoli, cauliflower, kale, Brussels sprouts and cabbage. You can experiment with the whole list of cruciferous vegetables: arugula, bok choy, broccoli, broccoli rabe, broccoli romanesco, Brussels sprouts, cabbage, cauliflower, Chinese broccoli, Chinese cabbage, collard greens, daikon garden cress, horseradish, kale, kohlrabi, komatsuna, land cress, mizuna mustard seeds and leaves, pak choi, radish, rutabaga, tatsoi, turnip root and greens, wasabi and watercress.

Also, at least twice a week include nutrient-rich energy-filled sprouts in your meals. The common ones You can find sunflower, mung-bean, radish, alfalfa and broccoli sprouts in most grocery stores. If you want to be more exotic, you can seek out delicious blends from specialty growers—Sprout People is famous for its "Bruno's Indoor Garden Micro-Greens Mix" of tatsoi, purple kohlrabi, red Russian kale, red cabbage, turnip, alfalfa, arugula, cress, red giant mustard, red oak and green romaine lettuce, mizuna, and pink and purple orach sprouts. Salads and sandwiches are the easiest ways to add sprouts to your meals, though you can go a step further and cook with them—for instance Asian, Middle Eastern, Indian and Mediterranean fusion dishes often include sprouts. Always thoroughly rinse sprouts under running water before eating.

SNACKS

Raw vegetables like cucumber slices, celery sticks and broccoli florets eaten alone or with a dip such as guacamole or tabouli are healthy alternatives to chips and popcorn. Or a plant-based smoothie with a dollop of almond butter added in, or just a spoonful of almond butter by itself, are other good choices. Hummus is a real winner too, especially with the explosion in creative blends with sun-dried tomato, spinach and artichoke, roasted garlic, chipotle, and roasted red pepper.

Enjoy it with carrot sticks, celery, a whole grain such as sprouted bread, or low-starch cracker like Mary's Gone Crackers.

A piece of fruit is an easy choice as well. An apple, pear, plum, or peach can be good on the go. Berries, too: blueberries, raspberries, strawberries and blackberries for instance. Just remember, only one serving per day of fruit and berries due to their natural sugars, and be especially moderate with the highest glycemic ones like bananas, grapes, apples, cherries, pears and dates.

Nuts of all varieties, except for peanuts, and seeds of all varieties in moderation are excellent go-to snacks. The best option is to choose unroasted, unsalted ones. Please don't let the fat content scare you away. As we discussed earlier, there are good fats and bad fats and several nuts, like almonds and walnuts, contain a lot of the good ones.

In a perfect world it would be best to close your kitchen down at 7 pm. But that's just not practical for most. It's important to know that your nighttime cravings are more often tied to the need for sleep and hydration than to the need for food. To be at your ideal weight and have the best night's sleep, slowly get used to going to bed just a bit hungry. Not so hungry that your stomach is screaming, but the emptier it is, the better. If you still need something more, drink a glass of water or unsweetened nondairy milk such as almond, soy, flax, or rice milk, or have a small serving of nuts, leftover pilaf, or piece of low-sugar fruit.

PUTTING IT ALL TOGETHER

HEALTH TAPESTRY MEAL PLAN

At a Glance

Please modify these suggestions for your particular allergies, tastes and dietary needs.

Leafy Green Veggies: Energy

Eat as many leafy greens as you like, especially raw ones, including as additions to smoothies. Tapestry favorites include spinach, kale, chard, greens and all kinds of lettuces.

Cruciferous Veggies: Protection

Popular ones include broccoli, cauliflower, arugula, Brussels sprouts and cabbage. Some are more digestible when slightly cooked.

Other Veggies: Diversity

Root veggies such as yams, carrots and beets are best eaten in moderation because of their high glycemic index; however, avoid white potatoes altogether. Some plant foods classified as veggies, like cucumbers and zucchini, are actually fruits, though they still are packed with high nutritional value and are low in calories.

Legumes: Balance

Chickpeas, lentils, most beans and peas are good sources of minerals and amino acids. Sprouts such as alfalfa, mung and clover are high-nutrient foods and a favored option in meal planning.

Nuts and Seeds: Strength

Raw and unsalted walnuts and almonds are the best nuts for healthy fat and protein. Many nut butters are great too. Super seeds include sunflower, sesame, flax, chia and raw and unsalted pumpkin seeds.

Whole Grains: Essentials

Top three favorite whole grains for nutritional value are buckwheat, quinoa and amaranth. They are gluten free, high in amino acids and rich in fiber.

Fruits: Treats

Low glycemic fruits like avocados, as well as plums and organic berries are Tapestry favorites, while high glycemic ones like bananas and grapes are best in moderation. Apples are high in fiber and filling, making them a go-to for dieters.

Dairy: Alternatives

Milk, yogurt and ice cream made from soy, almond, rice, oats and other plant foods are heart heathy, allergen-reduced dairy alternatives. However, they may contain high amounts of calories and sugar.

Olive Oil: Youthfulness

Extra-virgin olive oil is flavorful, heart-healthy and dense with anti-aging nutrients.

Plant Proteins: Wholeness

Tofu (soy) and tempeh (cultured soy); minimally processed plant-based burgers and loafs made with a blend of veggies, legumes and nuts; and smoothies made with pea, hemp or rice powders are great plant proteins for nutritional wholeness.

Meat: Moderation

Fresh fish in moderation, with limited amounts of organic eggs, poultry and lean grass-fed beef are healthy animal protein choices.

SUGGESTED WEEKLY MENU

The weekly menu that follows is intended to be a guideline. It is not meant to be a decree from on high. Eat the foods you like and skip the ones you don't. The wide variety of choices from our list gives you lots of flexibility to satisfy your tastes.

DAY 1

Breakfast: Either a plant-based smoothie such as Pro-Meal Advanced powder mixed with filtered water or almond, soy, flax or rice milk, or three to five ounces of a whole-grain pilaf. You can add a condiment such as Bragg Liquid Aminos or a dollop of a healthy butter alternative such as Earth Balance. Use a convenient blender bottle or a blender filled with ice and whatever greens you might have in the refrigerator—dark chocolate also goes well with milder tasting greens. We recommend choosing a consistent breakfast for most days of the week so it becomes a reflexive "go to" healthy routine.

Midmorning snack: ½ cup of blueberries.

Lunch: Green salad with three to six ounces of a protein such as a plant-based burger, tuna, or chicken breast. Top with extra-virgin olive oil and vinegar dressing, or freshly squeezed lemon juice.

Midday snack: Handful of almonds.

Dinner: Four- to six-ounce seared tempeh or salmon filet with lightly steamed broccoli that is then sautéed with garlic and extra-virgin olive oil.

DAY 2

Breakfast: Follow your routine from Day 1.

Midmorning snack: Toasted sprouted grain bread with almond butter or two rye crackers with hummus. Try Mary's Gone Crackers, which are made from whole grains, are low in starch and have gluten-free options.

Lunch: Mixed vegetables with sprouts salad. Top with extra-virgin olive oil, vinaigrette, or hummus.

Midday snack: Celery sticks and tabouli.

Dinner: Tofu vegetable stir fry with broccoli, bok choy and red onions over a bed of half a cup of quinoa pilaf. Quinoa is low in starch and has protein and good fat.

DAY 3

Breakfast: Follow your routine from Day 1.

Midmorning snack: One serving of soy, rice or other nondairy yogurt.

Lunch: Lightly steamed baby greens garnished with four ounces of tuna, topped with extra-virgin olive oil and lemon.

Midday snack: Vegetable smoothie blended with one apple, or a vegetable-based juice such as a drink-your-greens combination of spinach, cucumber, celery, lemon, ginger and apple.

Dinner: Roasted Brussels sprouts with shallots on a bed of lentil and brown-rice pilaf. Side salad with grated carrots, beets and parsnips seasoned with extra-virgin olive oil, balsamic vinegar and thyme.

DAY 4

Breakfast: Follow your routine from Day 1. Be adventurous and add fresh pumpkin to the pilaf or fresh ginger to the smoothie.

Midmorning snack: One apple.

Lunch: Chicken vegetable soup seasoned with fresh parsley and sage and a slice of sprouted bread.

Midday snack: Cucumber slices topped with hummus and mixed sprouts.

Dinner: Four- to six-ounce serving of Tuscan grilled trout with roasted Italian cauliflower seasoned with capers, tomatoes, oregano, basil and extra-virgin olive oil.

DAY 5

Breakfast: Follow your routine from Day 1.

Midmorning snack: Avocado spread on Mary's Gone Crackers Super Seed Seaweed & Black Sesame thins.

Lunch: Spinach, mushroom and tomato egg-white omelet.

Midday snack: Salsa and blue corn tortilla chips.

Dinner: Lightly steamed chopped asparagus combined with shiitake mushrooms sautéed in extra-virgin olive oil. Then plate on a bed of steamed cauliflower and millet and season with a sprig of sage and parsley.

DAY 6

Breakfast: Follow your routine from Day 1. Mix things up and add fresh walnuts or pecans.

Midmorning snack: One slice of sprouted grain bread. A glass of non-dairy, unsweetened almond, soy, flax or rice milk.

Lunch: Black bean soup. Side dish: jicama slaw and arugula, avocado and cilantro salad tossed in a vinaigrette.

Midday snack: Celery and carrot sticks with guacamole dip.

Dinner: Salad mix of lentil, pea, mung, adzuki and garbanzo bean sprouts tossed with extra-virgin olive oil, garlic, onion and spices. Side dish: four- to six-ounce serving of mild or spicy Sichuan tofu.

DAY 7

Breakfast: Follow your routine from Day 1.

Midmorning snack: One cup of raspberries.

Lunch: Miso soup with diced tofu. Side dish: stir-fried bok choy, chard, cabbage and other Asian vegetables.

Midday snack: Two handfuls of shelled, raw, unsalted sunflower seeds.

Dinner: Large spinach salad blended with bean sprouts, diced purple onion and mushrooms tossed with extra-virgin olive oil and lemon or a vinaigrette. Side dish: barley, wild rice and cranberry pilaf.

There's no shortage of great recipes to fit your tastes, but here are a few of our personal favorites:

DR. DAN'S TRAIL MIX

There are two different blends—one for men and one for women. The recipe for men contains pumpkin seeds, which are great for prostate health. The one for women contains flax seeds, which may provide support for menopausal symptoms.

Preheat the oven to 325 degrees.

In a large bowl mix:
1 pound raw almonds
1 pound raw walnuts
½ pound raw sunflower seeds (optional)
¼ pound organic raisins
a pinch of sea salt to taste
Men: add ½ cup of pumpkin seeds
Women: add ¼ cup of ground flax seeds
Some Like it Hot! If you like spicy food, sprinkle in a small amount of cayenne pepper.

Spread the trail mix on a baking sheet and drizzle on some Bragg Liquid Aminos seasoning. Cook for 10 to 15 minutes until mixture is lightly browned. Remove from oven. Enjoy warm or let it cool and store in a closed container.

DR. DAN'S EASY SALAD

Fresh herbs—four parts parsley to one part basil or sage

3 ounces extra-virgin olive oil

1 small fresh lemon

1 bag of organic mixed lettuce greens like baby spinach, mache and arugula

1 small ripe avocado

½ small onion or two shallots, finely chopped

1 plum tomato or four cherry tomatoes, diced

Dressing:

Soak the herbs in a large bowl with the olive oil for about 15 minutes, then squeeze the lemon juice in, lightly whip with a fork, and that's your dressing. Add all the other ingredients in a mixing bowl, toss with the dressing, and enjoy.

DR. ANTHONY'S SIMPLE SPROUT SALAD

This salad is delicious as a side dish with grilled salmon filet. Also, try it as a side with a vegetable stir-fry that has diced firm tofu, bok choy, snow peas, ginger and Bragg Liquid Aminos seasoning for an Asian fusion.

1 cup each of two or more different types of sprouts: alfalfa, barley, sunflower, mung bean, green lentil, broccoli, radish, clover, mustard

Extra-virgin olive oil

1 tablespoon of Bragg Liquid Aminos seasoning

2 brown rice cakes

Put sprouts in a large bowl, add enough olive oil to lightly coat them, and toss.

Add Bragg and mix again. If you like more of a soy-sauce taste, add more Bragg.

Crumble two brown rice cakes in the bowl, mix, and enjoy.

DR. ANTHONY'S PESTO ALL THE WAY FROM ITALY

1 bunch of basil leaves, no stems (can substitute spinach or parsley)

¼ cup of pine nuts (can substitute walnuts, pecans or a combination)

1 peeled garlic clove

Extra-virgin olive oil

Drop basil leaves, pine nuts and garlic clove into a food processor or blender.

Purée while slowly adding olive oil until desired consistency, and enjoy.

There is another aspect to eating well, and it is not so much about what you put in your mouth but rather what you put in your *mind*. In an upcoming chapter we will discuss more about the Marcus Institute of Integrative Health being at the forefront in the practice of mindfulness—the state of being aware, conscious, and in the present moment. Mindfulness has expanded beyond its roots to include nutrition and is referred to as mindful eating.

The benefits of applying mindfulness to eating are just as powerful as they are for other areas of your life. One exercise we recommend may sound silly because all you need to bring is a single raisin. "Raisin Meditation" is broken into five steps:

Hold, See and Touch: Examine your raisin closely. Look at its wrinkles, its colors. Is it squishy or hard? Puffy or dented? Does it feel sticky in your palm? Which ridges feel smooth and which sharp to your touch?

Smell: Lift the raisin to your nose and take in its fragrance. Does the sweet aroma make you salivate? Lick your lips? Take a deep breath? Does your stomach growl?

Place: Rest the raisin on your tongue. Just hold it there. Then draw it into your mouth and roll it around with your tongue without chewing. Can you sense the flavor changing as different taste buds are stimulated? How does the raisin feel against the roof and sides of your mouth? Is the raisin dissolving from your saliva?

Taste: Bite down on the raisin. Notice your jaw's movements. Notice the raisin's texture and flavor as you chew once. Then twice. Then three times, pausing between each bite to sense its sweetness, ridges and texture.

Swallow: Notice your throat muscles constricting and the position your tongue and jaw take as you prepare to swallow the raisin. Finally, swallow it.

This process slows you down, helps you savor the flavors, and gives you a sense of calmness. It also offers you a deeper understanding of your relationship with food that can translate into helping you unravel any tendencies toward overeating, eating out of frustration or boredom, binge eating, depriving yourself, and other emotional-based triggers. Another result is a healthier digestive system without competition for your attention from your television or computer. For an added bonus, invite someone you are close with to join you for a meal. If possible shop together, cook together, and make the whole meal an experience in mindful eating.

4

WEAVING IN WELLNESS WITH NUTRITIONAL SUPPLEMENTS

There are an estimated 100,000 beneficial phytonutrients in food, though we only have a limited understanding of a fraction of them. For example, a relatively new discovery indicates that consuming phytonutrient quercetin-rich foods such as apples and peppers can help improve cognitive functioning. A combination of the phytonutrients curcuminoid and piperine, found in turmeric and black pepper respectively, has been shown to have antioxidant properties to help slow the aging process.

"Great!" you might say. "But why bother with what's in the kitchen? I'll just go pick up a bottle of vitamins at the store." Good question. When a particular vitamin, mineral, enzyme, antioxidant or other phytonutrient is isolated and made into a pill, you miss out on the important sister compounds found in fresh whole food. Here's an example: When you eat an orange, you don't just get the vitamin C, you also get the full range of citrus bioflavonoids that are in the white-colored membranes of the inner peel. Eating a whole food often provides unique and synergistic health benefits that exceed what individual components have on their own. For instance, bioflavonoids can help reduce bruises.

To illustrate further, you can consume the same potassium, magnesium and vitamin C found in a peach in individual supplements. But by eating the fruit itself you get added value from peaches' four natural major phenolic compounds: anthocyanins, chlorogenic acids, quercetins and catechins that in combination help keep your weight in line. The fruit's phytonutrients also serve as prebiotics, which stimulate the growth of friendly bacteria in your intestines. So with this example that would mean taking a total of five supplements—potassium, magnesium, vitamin C, a digestive enzyme and acidophilus—to get close to the benefits from eating a fresh organic peach. And these are only five—so do you also take pills for the peach's glutathione, phenolics, delphinidin, rutin and carotenoids?

It is true a number of great supplement companies whose products consistently and reliably meet the highest quality standards include in their formulas a wide range of sister compounds like bioflavonoids, polyphenols (found in green tea), curcuminoids (found in turmeric), and mangiferin (found in mangoes) to name just a few. However, research shows the nutrients from natural foods are better absorbed and better utilized by the body than those from supplements.

As Aristotle said, "The whole is greater than the sum of its parts." Eating fresh food rather than depending on compartmentalized supplements builds on the synergy our integrative approach is founded on.

The conundrum, though, is that even if you eat well you may not get enough of some key nutrients. There are at least a few reasons we know of to help explain why this is so. Perhaps the main one is that food today is not what it used to be. In a study by Christian J. Charts entitled *Nutrient Changes in Vegetables and Fruits, 1951 to 1999,* the author concluded that a woman in 1951 who ate two peaches would have enough vitamin A for the day based on RDA guidelines. But today, that woman would need to eat 53 peaches to get the same amount of vitamin A.

A related seminal study by the University of Texas at Austin's Department of Chemistry and Biochemistry was published in the *Journal of the American College of Nutrition*. It concluded that soil depletion, pesticides, fertilizers and other additives designed to increase growth also have the unfortunate effect of decreasing the nutritional value of those crops. As you might imagine, advocates for organic farming have seized on these findings as further proof that conventional farming may be less expensive at the grocery checkout, but it is much more expensive overall when you take into account the costs associated with sickness. However, the nutrients in organic produce may not be enough either.

Another reason why eating fresh food alone may not be enough to meet your nutritional needs is the influence of harmful stress. What this means is if you live in a serene countryside, the spinach you eat is absorbed and utilized by your body better than the spinach you eat if you live in a big city. Furthermore, stress depletes your body of nutrients so you need a larger quantity to help offset the shortfall. One study using urine and hair analyses shows that people experiencing acute stress had an immediate loss of calcium, magnesium and zinc. Other studies showing that depletions of vitamins B, C and E, and minerals manganese, potassium and calcium due to stress corroborate these findings. This research highlights the importance of having a stress-reduction program, as we will discuss in the upcoming chapters.

The fact that most produce loses 30 percent of its nutritional value just three days after it is picked and the loss continues with each successive day, according to University of California studies, also helps explain why eating well may not be enough to give you the nutrients you need. Though the research is inconclusive, it appears that frozen options might be a reasonable second choice to fresh food, but canned foods definitely are not. For example, up to 95 percent of vitamin A, 72 per cent of vitamin C, and 50 percent of zinc typically disappears from canned mixed peas and carrots. In addition, research shows that while eating fresh vegetables has clear health benefits, eating canned ones may have the opposite effect.

Another well-documented reason why you may not get the nutrients you need just by eating fresh food has to do with the medicines you take. Research conducted by the Mayo Clinic shows that nearly 70 percent of Americans are on at least one prescription drug. Other research reveals that 93 percent of Americans commonly take nonprescription over-the-counter drugs. What you may not know is that many of these medications can deplete your body of important nutrients. Every time you pop an antacid, take medication to lower your blood pressure, or use an oral contraceptive, you increase your risk for vitamin B deficiency. B vitamins are not only good for your mood, well-being and heart health, they are also essential for driving natural chemical reactions inside the mitochondria of all of your cells to create the energy to run your body.

Below are examples of nutrient depletions from taking other widely prescribed drugs:

Thiazide Diuretics HCTZ for heart, liver and kidney disease

CoQ_{10}	Sodium
Magnesium	Zinc
Potassium	

Loop Diuretics for heart, liver and kidney disease

Calcium	Pyridoxine B_6	Vitamin C
Magnesium	Sodium	Zinc
Potassium	Thiamine B_2	

ACE (angiotensin-converting enzyme) inhibitors for high blood pressure

Sodium
Zinc

Beta Blockers for high blood pressure

CoQ_{10}
Melatonin

ARBs (angiotensin receptor blockers) for high blood pressure

Zinc

Centrally Acting Antihypertensives for high blood pressure

CoQ_{10}

HMG-CoA Reductase statins for high cholesterol

Carnitine	Essential Fatty Acids	Vitamin E
Copper	Selenium	Zinc
CoQ_{10}	Vitamin D	

Metformin for high blood sugar

CoQ_{10}

Folic acid

Vitamin B_{12}

In light of this, and certainly there's much more we don't yet know, we recommend a limited plan of daily supplements to help fill in any nutritional gaps. There are two important caveats though: 1) No amount of supplements can make up for a bad diet, and 2) Despite the continual barrage of false marketing, nutritional supplements cannot cure cancer. Once a cancer is diagnosed, conventional oncological care is necessary. However, good nutrition helps maintain a healthy body during the treatment process. A good diet might also help lower the risk of cancer recurrence.

The good news is you don't need to take a lot of supplements for optimal health. Personally, we keep our own regimens pretty simple and recommend the same for you: a multivitamin, omega-3 fatty acids, and a probiotic and prebiotic combination. We also recommend vitamin D_3 supplementation at about 2,000 IU daily.

There are a number of good supplement brands. If there is one you already like and it is working well for you, then by all means keep using it. Otherwise, we suggest you visit the Marcus Institute Online Store at https://marcusstore .jeffersonhealth.org/collections/shop for some of our recommendations. We do not receive any compensation from the store. It exists as a convenience for the patients we treat both here in our offices and via online appointments.

MULTIVITAMINS

Simplicity. This word is the strongest reason why a multivitamin is one of only four supplements we recommend for your daily plan. Antioxidants beta carotene and vitamins C and E; B-complex vitamins B_1, B_2, B_3, B_5, B_6, B_7, B_9 and B_{12}; essential minerals calcium, phosphorus, potassium and magnesium; trace minerals zinc, iron, copper, chromium and selenium—all in one dose—is just practical.

You can imagine how complicated and expensive it would be to take each of these as individual pills.

In addition to these basics, a good multivitamin will be formulated with compounds offering the highest absorption of nutrients, particularly minerals. Compounds to look for include citrates, palmitates and chelates versus carbonates, particularly in regard to minerals like calcium. The difference in pricing and bulkiness of the pills (or requirement to take several pills) often is due to these mineral complexes. The ones that are more easily absorbed tend to be bulkier molecules and more expensive.

Back-to-back reports of "The Physicians' Health Study II," published in the *Journal of the American Medical Association,* looked at whether there was an advantage to taking a daily multivitamin in terms of reducing risks for cardiovascular disease or cancer. These studies found that multivitamins did not offer an advantage for reducing cardiovascular disease. However, there was a modest but statistically significant benefit for protection against cancer. Overall, we did not find these results surprising. When it comes to cardiovascular disease, a primary dietary issue related to this condition is the excess of bad fats that cause systemic inflammation and plaque formation. A multivitamin may not help, but supplementing with omega-3 fatty acids has been shown to lower some of the bad fat such as triglycerides and LDLs. On the other hand, certain micronutrients are known to have a protective effect against gene mutations that lead to cancer. Results showing a benefit to having sufficient nutrients makes sense. Cancer is a multifactorial disease and highly complex, and other dietary factors play an important role in it as well. For example, being overweight and eating highly processed foods pose clear increased risks for cancer, but so do certain genetics and many other environmental factors such as pollution.

OMEGA-3 FATTY ACIDS

Omega-3s and omega-6s are essential fatty acids—*essential* being the operative word. Your body needs these good fats to run at optimal levels. The omegas are a major component of cell membranes—the protective covering that encases each of the trillions of cells in your body. The membranes' functions include allowing nutrients in and excreting waste out. They maintain the structural integrity of your cells and also serve as conduits through which communications between cells pass.

You more than likely get enough of—or even an excessive amount of—omega-6 in your diet from the foods you eat. It is in cooking oils, cereals, nuts and most other common foods. The reason to even think about them at all isn't so much deficiency but relative excess, especially compared to the healthier omega-3s. The key issue is that omega-6 contributes to inflammation whereas omega-3 is anti-inflammatory. Prior to industrialization the typical diet had an omega-6 to omega-3 ratio of somewhere between 1:1 and 4:1. Ideally that is what it would still be, but with all the cooking oils, processed foods, margarines, salad dressings, and more that people consume, the average American diet has skyrocketed to a ratio between 10:1 and 20:1!

Consuming enough omega-3 is very important. Let's go over some of the far-reaching implications. Omega-3 fatty acids are mainly broken down into two other fatty acids, eicosapentaenoic acid (EPA) and docosahexaenoic acid (DHA); though for our purposes you can simply use them interchangeably and consider them to be happily working beside each other. There are high levels of EPA and DHA in a healthy brain—correspondingly, low levels have been linked to depression, mental fogginess and Alzheimer's disease.

They are also shown to be important for cardiovascular health. In fact, the American Heart Association suggests omega-3s in part because they serve as anti-inflammatories, a benefit that has been associated with a reduced risk of coronary artery events including sudden heart attacks.

Omega-3s are commonly found in cold-water fatty fish—salmon, tuna, mackerel, halibut and sardines are the main ones—nuts, pumpkin seeds, flax seeds, some grains and a few other sources. However, it's difficult to get enough of them just from the food you eat.

For example, fish is the most popular source. But most of fish's omega-3 is concentrated in its skin, which many people don't eat. Fish do not "make" the omegas—they eat them in the algae at the bottom of the sea and concentrate them in their bodies. Another factor is whether the fish is wild or farm-raised. According to the Food and Agriculture Organization of the United Nations, 75 percent of salmon worldwide is farm-raised. That number is anticipated to increase as wild-caught salmon becomes more scarce and expensive. Farm processing techniques remove omega-3 fatty acids from the salmon to extend their shelf life at your grocery store, which is exactly what you don't want.

To have a good balance of omega-3s, we advise taking a daily supplement of 3,000 to 4,000 mg. There are two commercially viable sources for omega-3 supplements: fish and flax. Most of the studies confirming the health benefits of omega-3s have been performed using fish. For this reason, we recommend that you use a fish-based supplement, but be sure that it is certified by a third-party lab guaranteeing its purity. This guarantee of purity needs to be a deal breaker for you when deciding which brand to buy. That's because fish, like any living organism, interacts with its environment. It is vital that your supplement be free of mercury, polychlorinated biphenyls (PCBs), dioxins and other toxins. Labdoor, International Fish Oil Standards Program (IFOS), and Consumer Lab are among the most recognized third-party consumer watchdog guarantors of omega-3 purity. Look for their seals of approval. Store your fish oil omega-3 capsules in a cool, dark place out of direct sunlight.

Flaxseeds are the primary source of omega-3 fatty acid supplements for vegetarians. However, this form is not as easily absorbed by your body since it needs certain enzymes like delta-5, delta-6 desaturase and elongase for absorption. Unfortunately, in flax these enzymes do not always work well. You can still take a flax-based omega-3 supplement, but just be aware there is a debate about its effectiveness, and at this point it does not look favorable.

A note of caution: Omega-3 fatty acids are natural blood thinners. If you are taking a blood thinner in preparation for surgery, have a defibrillator or have other health considerations it is advisable to take omega-3 supplements only with the supervision of your treating physicians.

PROBIOTICS AND PREBIOTICS

Your gut is home to *trillions* of different microscopic organisms, collectively called the human microbiota, including hundreds of different species of "friendly" bacteria—also known as probiotics—such as Lactobacillus acidophilus, L. bulgaricus and B. bifidum, among others. You have an estimated ten times more bacteria in your gut than all the cells making up your entire body.

These friendly gut bacteria perform many crucial jobs. For example, they are essential to your digestive and immune systems, they work with your liver to clean out toxins, they help control the growth of bad bacteria, fungus and yeast; and they produce many vitamins, including three basic ones: B_{12}, folate and biotin. New research also shows they are essential to your emotional well-being and to maintaining optimal body weight.

In an article entitled "Nutritional Psychiatry: Your Brain on Food," Eva Selhub, MD and contributing editor at Harvard Health Publishing wrote: "Serotonin is a neurotransmitter that helps regulate sleep and appetite, mediate moods and inhibit pain. Since about 95% of your serotonin is produced in your gastrointestinal tract, and your gastrointestinal tract is lined with a hundred million nerve cells, or neurons, it makes sense that the inner workings of your digestive system don't just help you digest food, but also guide your emotions" by activating neural pathways from the gut to the brain and back.

This gut flora, plus your genetic makeup, determine a lot about your everyday health—for instance, when you step on the scale: the gut bacteria named Firmicutes store fats while Bacteroidetes burn them off. A lot of the former is linked to obesity while a lot of the latter is linked to leanness. Surely, your first swing at being healthy rested with having a healthy mother with a healthy flora. Her billions of good gut bacteria plus the 23,000 genes in your unique human genome combined to make you who you are today.

Aside from lifestyle, as we age our production of friendly bacteria tends to slow down, just like a lot of our other systems. Exposure to toxins, especially antibiotics, pesticides and pollutants also cuts into our probiotic supply. To help with your body's natural replenishment of these good bacteria, you can eat fermented foods such as sauerkraut, soy sauce, tempeh and kombucha. Yogurt is another food source for probiotics. However we don't recommend it or any dairy products—they are high in inflammatory fat and casein, and the amount of living cultures in commercial yogurts are relatively small.

Though clearly it's a nice idea to get as many probiotics from your diet as possible, there are questions as to whether enough active cultures are in the food we eat to make a real difference. That's why we recommend taking a probiotic supplement that contains multiple strains derived from non-dairy sources such as soy and rice. An ordinary dosage is 20 billion colony-forming units (CFUs) per day. To help support patients with specific inflammatory conditions we often recommend even larger dosages.

Moving on to prebiotics now, let's start with an analogy. Water is to your lawn what prebiotics are to your probiotics. Water nourishes your lawn to create your overall landscape. Prebiotics nourish your probiotics to create your overall gut microbiota.

If you don't water your lawn, you'll still have landscaping, but it won't be nearly as attractive. If you don't add prebiotics, you'll still have gut microbiota, but it won't be nearly as plentiful. Prebiotics are important to a maximally friendly gut bacteria colony. They help with both naturally occurring and disease-instigated changes in the composition, quantity and activity in your overall microbiota. A prebiotic that specifically increases the activity of friendly bifidobacteria and acidophilus-type organisms is best, along with general increases in any other friendly bacteria.

The gut surface of about 3,000 square feet is inhabited by 10 times the amount of bacteria than there are cells in the rest of the body. This means that besides the 23,000 genes of the human genome, we also live with a million bacterial genes. It is the combination of these two gene groups that makes us into who we are.

The gut wall is the encasement that surrounds the inside of the human body. That wall is what stands between us and death. It is a very thin wall and it must be protected at all costs. Its cells are united by special structures that resemble doors called tight junctions. They mostly remain closed and only open for specific reasons from the inside of the wall, such as to sample the outside environment for immune updates. If these doors open inappropriately, unchecked and unrefined materials from the hollow of the gut penetrate the bloodstream causing a calamity often referred to as leaky gut syndrome. The bloodstream, contaminated or clean, leads to one organ: the liver. Dirty substances that sneak into the blood supply and go to the liver are extremely disruptive.

The liver is commonly understood to be a wonderful, gigantic, friendly factory that builds all of the materials we need to survive. That is true, but the liver is also a weapon of war, sort of like an aircraft carrier loaded with airplanes, missiles, cannons, machine guns and explosives that when unleashed on the body create many ravaging diseases. It is not that the liver means to attack us; it does so when it mistakes the unrefined gut material contamination with our own bodies. This is likely how most autoimmune diseases start. You can think of this as friendly, but nonetheless deadly, fire as the contamination can have access to the whole body; to any place and any organ: skin, hair, lungs, kidneys, etc.

Many recent advances in science point to the notion that leaky gut may be a common link to a range of deadly diseases from a narrowing of the arteries to enlargement of the lymph nodes. Following this line of reasoning it becomes clear that preventing and healing leaky gut is a major objective in both preventing and healing disease. In our experience the three most important supplements to fix leaky gut are vitamin D$_3$, probiotics and prebiotics. That is partly why we advise them for everyone.

The right supplements can also help overcome bad genetics. Many people mistakenly believe that they can't do anything about their genes. This simply is not true. We all carry our fair share of good genes and bad genes. But here is the big news: they are not carved in stone. More precisely, genes have the potential to *express* (behave) differently in different situations. Genes tell the body how to build itself. They are the blueprint, and the machinery of life obeys those plans. Waking up genes that are harmful brings about the construction of a defective version of the body that could have been avoided by leaving them asleep.

Nutrition and lifestyle have the most powerful influence on gene expression and thus on what kind of body we have and build every day of our lives. So to a large extent much of our future is in our hands. This knowledge is so important! We make a point of teaching it to all of our patients.

For instance, there are different versions of the same gene which are called *polymorphisms*, and one version or another of them is activated by a person's lifestyle. It seems complicated but it helps explain what makes us unique. And it helps explain why it's possible for one brother to gorge on junk food and "get away with it" while the other can watch every morsel and still get into trouble.

An unhealthy lifestyle—smoking, being sedentary, eating poorly and having exposure to toxins—can activate harmful versions of genes. The good news is the reverse is also true: A healthy lifestyle can activate helpful genes and deactivate harmful ones, and the positive effect is magnified when combined with the right supplements. For example, a genetic predisposition toward anxiety could be stymied with a vitamin B complex supplement and an omega-3 fatty acid supplement, along with exercise and a low-sugar diet. Please see the brain imaging figures entitled Irritable Bowel Syndrome Treatment in the color photography section for evidence of the digestive system recovery that the Health Tapestry Meal Plan can offer.

VITAMIN D

Supplementation with Vitamin D, more accurately referred to as Vitamin D_3, has an interesting story. It's called the "sunshine vitamin" because we get this important nutrient directly from exposure to sunlight. Your grandparents likely never even gave a thought to vitamin D. After all, being outdoors was once a more typical part of American daily life.

But things have changed. Nowadays people are cautious about the sun's harmful UV rays and lather up with sunscreen and stay out of the sun more. Outdoor recreational activities have declined by nearly 25 percent in the last twenty years. The result is a staggering 85 percent of Americans are estimated to be deficient in vitamin D. We recommend 2,000 IU a day for most people. If you are fair skinned and okay with the idea of sun exposure, just ten minutes outdoors in midday several times a week might give you a sufficient level of Vitamin D without the need for further supplementation. If you are dark skinned then about two hours will likely do it. These amounts vary depending on the region you live in and the season.

PERSONALIZED SUPPLEMENTS

Our recommendation for a simple supplement plan composed of the four basics described above—a multivitamin, omega-3 fatty acids, a probiotic and prebiotic combination, and vitamin D3 —works great for most of our patients. Depending on your multivitamin and your lifestyle, you may also want to supplement with additional calcium. The recommended dosage for calcium is 1,000 mg a day for most people. If your multivitamin has 1,000 mg then you're covered. If it has 500 mg, you can add a 500 mg supplement to total the daily recommended 1,000 mg. Some calcium supplements have extra magnesium, which can be beneficial for greater nutrient absorption. In general, with vitamins and minerals you want to take into account your total daily consumption from all sources. For example, a cup of soy yogurt has 309 mg of calcium. A cup of cooked collard greens has 266 mg. What this means is if your multivitamin has 500 mg and you have soy yogurt for breakfast and collard greens for dinner then you will have reached the recommended 1,000 mg a day. Higher daily calcium intake is advised for women who are pregnant, over 50, or genetically predisposed to osteorosis.

We usually test our patients for specific conditions before recommending any additional supplements. Some of the most common ones among our optional add-ons are Nutritional shakes, CoQ10, and specific hormone balancers.

NUTRITIONAL SHAKES

We recommend nutritional shakes primarily for two groups: those who want to increase their nutritional intake, and those who use shakes as meal replacements because they want to healthfully reduce their caloric intake. There are some great plant-based formulations derived from high quality pea and rice protein. The most common one we recommend is Pro-Meal Advanced powder. For those trying to lose weight and balance blood sugar we use a similar product named Ultra Glucose Control® that has medium chain triglycerides (MCT) in it.

COQ$_{10}$

The naturally occurring antioxidant CoQ$_{10}$ has been well studied in clinical settings, specifically as part of treatment plans for high blood pressure and heart failure. But the statin drugs (e.g., Lipitor, Crestor, etc.) routinely prescribed for heart health can also decrease CoQ$_{10}$ production. In addition, CoQ$_{10}$ levels decline naturally with aging. Supplementation has been shown to increase physical well-being, and also male fertility. We recommend an ordinary dosage of 60 to 100 mg daily. Other dosages are best taken under the supervision of a knowledgeable physician.

HORMONE BALANCERS

Although genetics play an important role in hormone metabolism, diet plays an equal if not more important role. For example, many fruits and vegetables contain phytochemicals that can help improve hormone metabolism, which might explain why people who eat plant-based diets have the lowest rates of cancer. However, once there is an imbalance, it is difficult to normalize it with diet alone. The best of these supplements will also support overall health, weight control and vitality.

In our own study on hormones, alongside our colleagues Drs. George Zabrecky and Andrew Newberg here at the Marcus Institute of Integrative Health, conducted with middle-aged women to determine if estrogen ratios could be positively influenced by taking the multi-nutrient supplement product we designed called Lucentia Peak for Her®, the results showed a clear and significant increase in positive hormonal ratios. Healthier ratios have been shown to correlate with an improvement in estrogen metabolism and a reduced risk for gynecological cancer.

Lucentia Peak® has more than ten specialty nutrients. Three of them—calcium-D-glucarate, DIM (diindolylmethane), and resveratrol—are especially important:

The detoxifier calcium-D-glucarate is a naturally occurring substance produced in the body and found in many fruits and vegetables, especially cruciferous vegetables such as broccoli, cauliflower and Brussels sprouts. Supplementing accelerates detoxification.

The naturally occurring hormone stabilizer DIM (diindolylmethane) is also found in cruciferous vegetables. Supplementing increases the ability to regulate hormonal biological properties including changing harmful estrogen to helpful estrogen.

Hormone normalizer resveratrol is a naturally occurring phytoestrogen found in red grapes, red wines, berries and peanuts, among other foods. Supplementing improves ability to restore balanced hormone levels and slow down aging.

Please visit Lucentia at www.mylucentia.com for more information. Disclaimer: We designed this product and have a direct affiliation with it.

For further information on some of our other studies that have helped establish our team as international experts on the use of natural molecules such as ascorbic acid (Vitamin C), N-Acetyl Cysteine (NAC) in patients with cancer, Parkinson's disease and other conditions, please see the brain imaging figures entitled Parkinson's Disease Treatment in the color photography section, as well as the following publications:

Monti, Daniel A., Edith Mitchell, Anthony J. Bazzan, Susan Littman, George Zabrecky, Charles J. Yeo, Madhaven V. Pillai, Andrew B. Newberg, Sandeep Deshmukh, Mark Levine: "Phase I Evaluation of Intravenous Ascorbic Acid in Combination with Gemcitabine and Erlotinib in Patients with Metastatic Pancreatic Cancer." *PLoS ONE* 7 no. 1, (2012).

Rouleau, Lauren, Anil Noronha Antony, Sara Bisetto, Andrew Newberg, Cataldo Doria, Mark Levine, Daniel A. Monti, Jan B. Hoek: "Synergistic effects of ascorbate and sorafenib in hepatocellular carcinoma: New insights into ascorbate cytotoxicity." *Free Radical Biology and Medicine*, 95 (June 2016): 308-322.

Monti, Daniel A., George Zabrecky, Daniel Kremens, Tsao-Wei Liang, Nancy A. Wintering, Jingli Cai, Xiatao Wei, Anthony J, Bazzan, Li Zhong, Brenden Bowen, Charles M. Intenzo, Lorraine Iacovitti, Andrew B. Newberg: "N-Acetyl Cysteine May Support Dopamine Neurons in Parkinson's Disease: Preliminary Clinical and Cell Line Data." *PLoS ONE*, 11 no. 6 (June 2016): e0157602. DOI:10.1371/journal.pone.0157602, 2016.

Monti, Daniel A., George Zabrecky, Daniel Kremens, Tsao-Wei Liang, Nancy A. Wintering, Anthony J. Bazzan, Li Zhon, Brenden K. Bowens, Inna Chervoneva, Charles Intenzo, Andrew B. Newberg: "N-Acetyl Cysteine Is Associated with Dopaminergic Improvement in Parkinson's Disease." *Clinical Pharmacology & Therapeutics*, 106 vol. 4 (October 2019):884-890

5

WEAVING IN MIND-BODY TRANSFORMATION

As we discussed earlier, unhealthy foods, excess body fat, poor sleep and lack of exercise can all increase inflammation. But there is another big source of inflammation: stress. Each of us has our own mind-body biosystem, and how we perceive life events and the world around us and then react to them can have a significant impact on the rest of our physiology and biochemistry. In fact, stress levels left unchecked can wreak havoc throughout your body and open doors to disease.

Our hardwired stress responses and all of their offshoots have a good side for sure. They motivate us to keep us safe and alive, whether to meet an important deadline or to flee from a lion in the jungle. That is what we call "good stress." But even a good stress response is designed to be short lived so that we switch it off to a relatively unstressed state. There's the catch—the switch often gets stuck in the "on" position. The lions of our evolutionary past are replaced today by an unrelenting boss, a sick parent, a struggling child, and so on. For many of us, just as one stressor subsides another starts, and we are frequently juggling several stressors all at once.

This kind of constant distress is unequivocally, quantifiably bad—actually more than bad. Bad stress is a major factor in the six leading causes of death in the United States: cancer, coronary heart disease, accidental injuries, respiratory disorders, cirrhosis of the liver and suicide. The Centers for Disease Control and Prevention estimates that stress accounts for about 75 percent of all US doctor visits while the Occupational Health and Safety Administration reports that number could be as high as 90 percent.

Fortunately, we have integrative solutions. Stress is not just a mental state; *it's a whole-body experience*. It can pervade all aspects of your health and well-being, leaving you depleted physically and emotionally.

Your body's response to stress is controlled by a branch of your nervous system called the *autonomic* nervous system (ANS). This system also controls the functions of many different organs, regulates heartbeat, controls breathing and aids digestion. The best, and worst, part is that your ANS does this all without you having to think about it—stress is perceived as some kind of threat to your well-being which causes the ANS to go into "fight-or-flight" mode. The overall response mechanism is the same whether you are running late to catch a flight at the airport or running from a lion to keep from getting eaten. It is just the intensity of the stress response that varies depending upon how bad the threat is perceived to be. Here's how it unfolds:

First, in response to whatever the threat is, your ANS orders a series of physiological reactions that rev up your body. Your adrenal glands pump higher levels of stress hormones, such as adrenaline and cortisol, into your bloodstream. Your kidneys release renin, a hormone that raises your blood pressure. Your heart pumps faster. Blood is pulled away from your midsection, thereby slowing down gut functions. Your blood sugar soars. Your pupils dilate so you can see better. Your immune cells spew out inflammatory chemicals to stop bleeding and fight infection in case either occur. In general, you gear up to fight or run for your life.

Now imagine what happens when this condition is chronic and your body is perpetually in a state of bad stress: you have an increased risk for high blood pressure, cardiac disease, poor sugar metabolism, digestive problems, difficulty sleeping, poor immunity and susceptibility to illness, to name just a few issues. Sound familiar?

It doesn't stop there. In the brain, high levels of stress hormones are associated with imbalances in neurotransmitters such as serotonin, norepinephrine and dopamine that allow your brain cells to regulate your mood and behavior. An imbalance of these chemicals—too much of one or too little of another—can lead to depression and anxiety. Bad stress can also affect levels of the amino acid homocysteine which, when elevated, can increase the risk for Alzheimer's disease and stroke.

Bad stress can also affect your sex life, both directly and indirectly. When you are in stress mode, you're thinking about survival, not sex. This makes sense from an evolutionary point of view—when our prehistoric ancestors were running from predators, their brains' focus shifted to the best ways to escape. Furthermore, when you're in stress mode the adrenal gland's contribution to sex hormones shuts down in favor of putting that energy into fight-or-flight. The overall results are fewer sex hormones, a lower libido and an inability to perform.

In your everyday life you probably most commonly experience bad stress as anxiety. From there it usually goes in two directions: you turn your stress inward—for instance, shovel down food to soothe yourself, engage in some addictive behavior, ruminate, or veg out in front of the television—or you turn it outward against others—for instance, look for fights, drive with road rage, or lash out.

At its root, the answer lies in emotional regulation. Emotional regulation boils down to being aware of your emotions and having effective tools to navigate them. How best to go about that is a subject of great debate. Based on our own studies and the findings of extensive research from around the world, we have found that an integrative approach is as effective for emotional wellness as it is for nutrition as described in our Health Tapestry Meal Plan.

It is no coincidence that new research keeps revealing more about the food/emotion connection. In particular, short chain fatty acids (SCFA) found in vegetables, fruits and legumes are extremely important for healthy emotional functioning. One exciting breakthrough from understanding this cause and effect relationship is a new area of study known as nutritional psychiatry. Nutritional psychiatrists study how consuming certain foods physically reshape the brain—most notably by reducing and preventing inflammation. In relation to emotional well-being, inflammation is linked to causing depression. The typical American diet is to inflammation what a bee is to honey. In effect, we help produce our own depression. We have a 25 to 35 percent higher risk of depression than those with a Japanese or Mediterranean diet rich in plant-based foods like vegetables, fruits, nuts and whole grains, as well as fish, and little, if any, meat or dairy; and no processed or refined foods.

One recently published report suggests a mechanism that may help explain this fact. Plant fiber-rich foods travel to the colon and feed both the cells of the colon and the healthful microbiome. They in turn produce the SCFAs from the food and send them directly to the brain via the general circulatory system. However, processed, refined foods never make it to the colon; they enter the body via the small intestine and create obesity and inflammation. The proper colon bacteria, and consequently the brain, are then left begging for SCFAs to help with healthy emotional functioning.

The Tapestry Mind-Body Transformation Plan also focuses on the ways you perceive life events and then react to them. This approach addresses the fundamental necessity to regulate your emotional processing through self-acceptance and through nourishing your emotional health. This can take a lifetime to master, but big transformations can come quickly with some focused attention, patience and TLC. In the words of the great vocalist Lena Horne, "It's not the load that breaks you down, it's the way you carry it."

You are probably already doing things to self-regulate your emotions without even realizing it. For example, do you ever take in a deep breath and let out a heavy sigh before you say something you're uncomfortable with? Do you ever throw your hands up in the middle of a disagreement, shake your head and walk away without saying anything? These are both common instances of slowing down the process by even a nanosecond to help transform your hurt and pain into comfort and grace. On the opposite side are all of the times you and every one of us loses it; represses; self-medicates; gets headaches, seeks distractions, and more.

A word about distractions: heaven knows we have enough of them now to last a lifetime. Between the internet, 24/7 news cycles, work-to-death ethos, and a shop-till-you-drop culture, there are plenty of opportunities to procrastinate, deny and bury our emotions. But if we could distract ourselves to emotional well-being then we'd all be living in a Golden Age. Instead, the more we rely on avoidance, the more we find ourselves in a Golden Cage. Smothered with the allure of the newest iPhone, the latest YouTube sensation, luxuries and bargains, followers and likes, you can easily go down these rabbit holes looking for relief from your stressful life but won't ever find it there. At least not relief that lasts.

For relief that lasts, we offer two main approaches in our program: Mindfulness and the Neuro Emotional Technique (NET). This in no way implies that they are the only two effective approaches, but they are the ones we use with our patients, the ones we have researched extensively, and the ones we use ourselves.

MINDFULNESS

The Marcus Institute at Jefferson offers the largest number of mindfulness-based programs of any medical facility in the country. Our model was developed from Jon Kabat-Zinn's Mindfulness-Based Stress Reduction (MBSR) approach and has been systemized into a formal stress reduction program as well as adapted for special situations. We also recommend his books, including *Full Catastrophe Living* and *Wherever You Go There You Are.*

Mindfulness means learning to objectively *pay attention* to your inner dialogue in the present moment, essentially, creating the mental clarity to look at "what is" rather than "what could have been" or "what should be." Strengthening your "observer self" as it is often called affords you more opportunities to make better choices. To enhance your observation of the present moment, our other mindfulness programs teach calming techniques and meditative exercises, some of which are grounded in the basic principles of yoga.

The overall process of building mindfulness can become quite complex, which is one reason why we strongly recommend doing as much training as possible, including enrolling in a well-researched full mindfulness-based program. In keeping with our overall philosophy of making a healthy lifestyle widely accessible, we have simplified some of our mindfulness training into a daily basic 20- to 30-minute two-step plan, and offer some optional add-ons.

The first step is to spend time each day just observing your thoughts and feelings without casting any judgments. None whatsoever. For instance, if you have thoughts like *I really blew it in that meeting* or *I scored big time in that meeting,* acknowledge, accept and move on. No need for self-berating or self-congratulating, for worrying or fantasizing. This is the first step to knowing yourself better and to having greater self-awareness. Essentially, you create the space to look at "what is," which affords you the opportunity to better choose your reactions.

The second step is to breathe. You may be thinking, "I already breathe just fine," but the truth of the matter is that like many of us, you likely spend most of the day in choppy breathing patterns. Volumes of independent research from around the world show that simply changing your breathing patterns can help melt stress. When you're in a fight-or-flight response, you tend to take short, shallow breaths, and even hold your breath for moments at a time. But by deliberately lengthening and deepening your breathing you can break this pattern and calm yourself down.

Maintaining endless rhythmic breathing—a gentle inhale to gentle exhale to gentle inhale around and around—over a lifetime is the ideal; admittedly that is one ideal few of us ever come close to achieving, let alone even attempting. That's why we offer an approach that takes much less commitment, but offers almost immediate benefits.

Five minutes is a good amount to begin with, if you have the time. If you don't, two minutes is still enough to help you feel calmer and more focused. To get started, we recommend you take at least two breathing breaks a day; one in the morning and another in the afternoon or evening. Some people find taking the second one in the afternoon helps re-energize them, while others find taking it in the evening helps them wind down before bedtime. Feel free to increase to three or more breathing breaks. See what works best for you as you follow the seven easy steps below, knowing that much like muscles in your body strengthen with exercise, your rhythmic breathing strengthens with exercise too. You will likely be pleasantly surprised at what a huge difference a couple of minutes a day makes.

1. Sit in a comfortable position. Try to clear your mind. This is your time, your break. Don't let intrusions in during your few-minute escape.

2. Take in a deep breath. Focus on your inhalation. Feel the air travel into your lungs and your stomach. It is best to breathe through your nose, if possible (both inhalations and exhalations). Fill your lungs, but do so comfortably without forcing the air.

3. Concentrate on releasing your breath. Feel the air traveling from your stomach up through your chest to your nose and out. It may be helpful to count four full seconds for the inhale and six seconds for the exhale.

4. Keep breathing in and out rhythmically, thinking about how naturally and effortlessly your lungs are filling up and emptying.

5. Be aware of how your deep breathing feels throughout your body. Notice how your muscles relax, how tension eases in your gut.

6. If your mind starts to wander, if you find yourself thinking about unrelated or even stress-provoking things, that's normal. Just observe them without judgment and gently reset your thoughts so that you once again become focused on your breathing.

7. Toward the end of your two to five minutes, when you're down to your last few breaths, end each one with a relaxing sigh or "Ahhh" sound. It's fine if you like another sound better such as "Om."

That's it. Those are the two basics: observe and breathe. Spending just 20 to 30 minutes a day practicing mindfulness and another two to five minutes a couple of times a day doing focused breathing can be really transformative. If you want more than this you can enroll in a full mindfulness-based program. The Marcus Institute even offers some online programs you can take from home—for more information please visit www.marcusinstitute.jeffersonhealth.org.

There are some wonderful add-ons if you want more than the basics. For instance, as a part of building your mindfulness, we suggest the "loving kindness" meditation. Below is an adaptation of it from *Teaching Mindfulness: A Practical Guide for Clinicians and Educators*, co-authored by Diane Reibel, director of the Marcus Institute's mindfulness programs:

In loving kindness meditation you set an intention to nurture the quality of the loving kindness that already exists within you while being without judgment about whatever is present in your senses, thoughts and emotions. By practicing loving kindness meditation you can become more familiar with this quality so that it is easier to recognize and become more spontaneously available to cultivate for yourself and for others. Just like mindfulness, this approach is a life-long commitment, an investment of time and energy that delivers immeasurable value. If any part does not suit you, please feel free to change it to be more friendly for you.

LOVING KINDNESS MEDITATION

Take a comfortable posture to enter your meditation, feeling your body where it makes contact with the support beneath you, settling in, centering yourself by focusing on your breath.

Think of someone easy for you to feel loving kindness toward: perhaps a friend, a child, a pet, a simple relationship.

Hold them in your awareness, seeing them in your mind's eye or feeling a sense of them in your heart.

As you hold them in your awareness, begin to send them wishes of loving kindness by silently repeating these phrases:

May you be peaceful and happy
May you be safe from harm
May you be as healthy and strong as you can be
May you live with the ease of well-being

When you are ready, allow this sense of them to fade.

Think of yourself as someone to feel loving kindness toward. Hold your awareness on seeing yourself in your mind's eye or feeling a sense of yourself in your heart.

As you hold your awareness, begin to send yourself wishes of loving kindness by silently repeating these phrases:

May I be peaceful and happy
May I be safe from harm
May I be as healthy and strong as I can be
May I live with the ease of well-being

Hold the intention of loving kindness toward yourself, even if it feels artificial, stilted, or you are not feeling any loving kindness in the moment.

Begin again to send yourself wishes of loving kindness by silently repeating these phrases:

May I be peaceful and happy
May I be safe from harm
May I be as healthy and strong as I can be
May I live with the ease of well-being

Begin again to outwardly send loving kindness to someone else by silently repeating these phrases:

May you be peaceful and happy
May you be safe from harm
May you be as healthy and strong as you can be
May you live with the ease of well-being

As you hold them in your awareness, continue to send them wishes of loving kindness by silently repeating these phrases:

May you be peaceful and happy
May you be safe from harm
May you be as healthy and strong as you can be
May you live with the ease of well-being

Be aware that the heart has its seasons, and feelings cannot be forced. Be as you are, aware of rising feelings, free of all judgments.

Expand the intention of loving kindness to simultaneously include yourself and others: those you know well and those you know less well; those you love and those you love less; and those around the world you will not ever meet.

As you hold yourself and them in your awareness, send wishes of loving kindness by silently repeating these phrases:

May we all be peaceful and happy
May we all be safe from harm
May we all be as healthy and strong as we can be
May we all live with the ease of well-being

Begin again to send wishes of loving kindness by silently repeating these phrases:

May we all be peaceful and happy
May we all be safe from harm
May we all be as healthy and strong as we can be
May we all live with the ease of well-being

Be with yourself as you are in the moment.

When ready, bring your attention back to feeling your body where it makes contact with the support beneath you, settling in, centering yourself by focusing on your breath.

Emerge gently from your meditation. Continue to be with yourself as you are in the moment, without judgment about whatever is present in your senses, thoughts and emotions—this in and of itself is an act of loving kindness.

Journaling is another way to complement your mindfulness practice. We suggest that at the end of each day you write down the main thoughts you told yourself during the day, both the nice thoughts and ugly ones. This requires not only paying attention to the dialogue going on inside your head, but also to observing and expressing it.

Another journaling approach is to focus on specific emotions you are experiencing. If you are feeling sad, for example, describe the sensation. Do the same with joy, anger, fear and the rest. Accept them all without favoritism. If you don't enjoy writing, you can have the same benefits by talking out loud and even recording your words, or drawing, sketching or painting. In fact, a combination of these can have a big impact on your life.

Along with our colleagues at Jefferson, in 2006 we published a study entitled "A Randomized, Controlled Trial of Mindfulness-based Art Therapy (MBAT) for Women with Cancer" in the medical journal *Psycho-Oncology*, which showed tremendous results. We followed up on this with an extensive study that revealed the superiority of this mindfulness intervention and standard support together over standard support alone in female cancer survivors. Our findings were published in 2013 in *Psycho-Oncology* under the title "Psychosocial Benefits of a Novel Mindfulness Intervention Versus Standard Support in Distressed Women with Breast Cancer." Further, we demonstrated impressive results in brain scans, showing positive activation of the executive functioning part called the pre-frontal cortex and positive deactivation of the impulsive fight-or-flight part called the amygdala. Please see the brain imaging figures entitled Breast Cancer Therapy in the color photography section for evidence of these results. That companion study was published in 2013 in the medical journal *Stress & Health* under the title "Changes in Cerebral Blood Flow and Anxiety Associated with an Eight-week Mindfulness Program in Women with Breast Cancer."

It is important to note that constructively owning your feelings is very different from destructively acting out impulses. Potential actions connected to tumultuous feelings would be best expressed first in the privacy of your journal. When you accomplish a sense of reconciling with yourself, then you have a clearer path to reconciling with others. There's a catch though: it requires patience. When you put in the effort to understand the bigger picture of your emotional life, you develop a greater sense of control over the direction of your whole life.

The Tapestry Mind-Body Transformation Plan is grounded in a scientific understanding of the emotional or *feeling* part of the brain and the logical or *thinking* part of the brain as being in distinct anatomical regions with distinct neurological pathways. These two parts of the brain can easily become disconnected, which is why you sometimes feel one way and think another: *I feel angry they didn't ask for my opinion in the meeting,* even while you're logically thinking *why would they? I don't know anything about that topic.*

The real problem is that the emotional part of the brain reacts faster than the thinking part, so you get upset before you have time to think things through. A primary reason for this disconnect is the fight-or-flight mode we've talked about, plus the evolution-based survival mechanisms that go along with it that push more adaptive responses further away. But just like learning any new skill, with practice and reinforcement you can "unlearn" the old and replace it with the new. The more you can counter much of the fight-or-flight mode with mindfulness, exercise, spirituality, rest, journaling and other mind-body interventions, the more your thoughts and emotions will be in balance and the better your quality of life will be.

Another exercise we suggest to accomplish a better congruence between thoughts and feelings is to focus on a specific situation. For example, think about a person who is a source of great stress for you—maybe it's your boss or a family member, or someone who's taken advantage of you. When you think about them, ask yourself, *What am I saying to myself about this person?* Write your response down after you say it out loud. Then ask, *What am I saying to myself about myself in regard to this person?* Write this response down too after you say it out loud. Framing your situation as a question, saying the answer out loud, and then writing down the answer can be an effective way to connect the feeling and thinking parts of your brain that allows for some neurological communication that was previously shut off. After you've finished your foundational questions, you can move on to some advanced ones like: *Is it possible for me to see this person differently? Is it possible for me to see this person's perspective, even if I think my perspective is right?*

Your first reaction to getting your thoughts and feelings to become friends might be: "Seriously? That's like pop psychology or religion or something." But please keep in mind that we are approaching this from the vantage point of science, not religion, though they may overlap. Our goal is not to convert you, it's to inform you that more balanced neurology leads to more happiness. Incidentally, it also allows for better engagement with personal spirituality if you so choose, or for more harmony with the world around you, which some would argue is spiritual in itself.

After looking at your internal dialogue about the world around you, sometimes you might find that the issue isn't an exaggerated internal response but that your negative reaction is a healthy alarm to something actually dangerous, like a deceitful person. Mindfulness and the other strategies we've suggested can strengthen your ability to decide which reactions are appropriate and which are not, and can help you respond to external circumstances in ways that work best for you. Sometimes this can lead to insights that will make relationships better, but sometimes it can lead to insights that will reveal relationships that must either be fixed or let go of.

Another activity we suggest is taking time to reflect upon and express your gratitude for anything and everything that is good in your life. Doing this has powerful neurological benefits because it establishes a connection between a thoughtful assessment and an especially powerful emotional state. The scientific research behind this is also an important component in the new and empirically supported field of Happiness Psychology. Gratitude has been revealed to be an essential element of happiness, along with having a sense of purpose and of community.

As part of your journaling, you can apply your expression of gratitude toward improving your relationships. Write down three things you appreciate about your partner, friend or family member, and another three things you appreciate about your relationship together. This not only helps you stay connected with the important aspects of your bond, it is also a good tool to have handy when navigating the ups and downs that are a normal part of any close relationship.

All of these suggestions ask you to take a bit of time to unwind with yourself every day. Yes, we know self-care has gotten a bad rap in some circles. Baby Boomers have been nicknamed the "Me Generation" and Millennials the "Me Me Me Generation." But there is not a fine line between selfishness and self-care—there's a wide chasm between the two. Extravagant self-indulgence and only experiencing things that are pleasurable in order to avoid discomfort are actually the opposite of self-care. The reality is we live in a world that is fraught with challenges, and our hope is to best navigate through these things internally and externally to give us the greatest satisfaction in life possible.

While self-indulgence certainly is an issue for some, many people have the opposite problem. Taking time for yourself is critical, and it's a natural and necessary part of mind-body wellness. Beyond practicing mindfulness, meditating, journaling, and more, we each need time to cultivate our nourishing emotions—the big three are interest, excitement and joy. There are numerous synonyms for these three; for instance, one of our patients likes to substitute the word joy for "happy place." Whatever words you like best for the distinct emotional states these three emotional categories trigger is fine. These emotions soothe us and counter the harmful effects of the emotions that drain us. How to make this spark happen is different for everyone.

As an example, you can take a day to do absolutely nothing but enjoy the garden in your backyard, listen to your favorite music, stay in your pajamas and read a book, or whatever it is that will evoke pleasurable emotions for you. We suggest you carve out some time at least once a week to do whatever replenishes you. The essence of self-care is that *you* make the rules. You keep them and you change them as you wish, as long as you give them top priority in your daily life.

Lastly, let's talk about socializing. We are hardwired to thrive on social connections—there is plenty of research showing how isolation negatively impacts our health. Unfortunately, as a society our sense of connection is becoming more fragmented. This collapse started before Facebook and Instagram, before "likes" and "tweets," though social media has made the situation worse for some.

The fact is, our culture has changed dramatically since World War II when the traditional nuclear family was the structure for developing community ties. Through a variety of economic and social changes the overall fabric of the American family has transformed, and for many this has led to isolation. The old ways of socializing, such as through neighborhood gatherings or religious organizations, are not as common today. Your career or other personal reasons may have moved you far away from your family of origin but you haven't established a surrogate family through a community. Despite the breakneck pace of the changes and challenges of modern life, stripped down, sincere face-to-face connections are a necessary part of personal fulfillment—they are a part of your neurological health.

This means you may have to try harder to make social connections than previous generations did, but nevertheless you have to do it for your own well-being and that of your community. It could be through a civic group, a sports team, a political organization, a book club—what is crucial is that you feel you belong and have nice people in your life. If you've moved away from your old group of friends, certainly it's good to stay connected with them, but at the same time it is also important to put yourself out there and make new ones. Having light moments of sharing laughter nourishes the soul and has been shown to have a healing effect on the body and mind. Quoting the twentieth century philosopher Kahlil Gibran from his book *The Prophet*, "And in the sweetness of friendship let there be laugher and sharing of pleasures. For in the dew of little things the heart finds its morning and is refreshed."

NEURO EMOTIONAL TECHNIQUE (NET)

In the mid-1980s, a young chiropractor named Scott Walker was on a mission to better understand why some of his patients did not maintain the physical adjustments that he had spent years mastering. He believed that nutrition likely played a role and that energy as understood by Chinese medicine factored in, but he was convinced there was something else, too.

His "a-ha" moment came while watching a demonstration of a woman who had been in a car accident and who had been having a difficult time maintaining chiropractic correction ever since. Her chiropractor had her visualize the moment of the accident while adjusting her. Lo and behold, this had a dramatic effect— she not only felt better, but the chiropractic adjustment finally held.

From there Dr. Walker began exploring how emotional events affected the body's ability to heal. His research included consideration of psychological concepts like "repetition compulsion" that Sigmund Freud had worked on some sixty years earlier. Freud's theory essentially said that unresolved emotions live on and erupt repetitively in often tangential but nevertheless significant maladaptive behaviors. Dr. Walker also explored the psychophysiological literature related to the many ways the body gives objective feedback when there is a perceived stressor, and considered Pavlov's experiments showing that responses to cues can be conditioned.

All of this led Dr. Walker to organize a revolutionary set of principles into a several-step procedure to identify distressing emotional events that impede an individual's mind-body system in some way, and then to resolve them. His process, the Neuro Emotional Technique (NET), aims to find and unwind conditioned response patterns with the goal of freeing patients to live healthier, happier lives. That was certainly the case with one of our patients.

At 55 years young, Harold was diagnosed with stage III colorectal cancer. It was a long road back, but he made it with the care of an excellent oncology team;

three years later he was still cancer-free. "A bullet dodged," he and his family said thankfully.

It turned out his body had dodged, but his psyche had not, as he continued to suffer from irritability, poor concentration and depression. Being a cancer survivor, he learned, was more than beating carcinomas. He was still in a fight against stress—or more accurately for him, distress.

The distress he showed even three years after his cancer treatments caused us to look deeper. He was quite willing, even emphatic, that having had cancer was behind this "mess." He described the day his doctor gave him the diagnosis as the "worst day of my life." He said he could barely hear anything after that as his mind raced: *I'll be dead soon and won't have time to get things in order. Who's going to look after my aging mother? I'm not going to know my grandchildren.* The more he talked about the "hell I went through," the more animated and agitated he became, as if he was reliving it in that moment. Finally, he had to stop. It was all too real.

It became clear that yes, the treatments for his cancer were stressful, but the moment at which he was told he had cancer is when he really became unhinged. Harold revealed that his father, with whom he was quite close, had died of the same type of cancer about twenty-two years before. He remembered how much his dad had suffered and how quickly he had deteriorated. So when Harold received the same diagnosis as his father, he was sure he'd have the same fate. We asked him to rate how distressing it had been to hear his diagnosis, using a scale from zero to ten with zero being no distress and ten being the highest level of distress imaginable. He answered, "Eleven."

Over the previous several years, the Marcus Institute had already built a good track record with the Neuro Emotional Technique (NET) for treating patients who had suffered from traumatic or distressing events. Fortunately, Harold was able to continue that streak after receiving NET treatment, and went on to live a fuller life; still cancer-free.

Dr. Walker and his wife Dr. Deb Walker have since refined the NET protocol over the years to address mind-body physiology through a combination of chiropractic philosophies, leading-edge psychological principles, focused breathing and ancient Chinese medicine pulse points.

Most of us have suffered from traumatic events in our lifetimes. You may have experienced a health scare, divorce, or death of a loved one. You may have been deeply humiliated, bullied, or failed at a crucial task. Often these events resolve themselves soon after they occur because you have the resources and mind-body reserves to do so. Other times they continue to live on, weigh down your quality of life, and trap you in ways you may not realize. NET provides a way out of this—it's not the only way, but it's the one we have found to be most efficient and effective.

In the prestigious *Journal of Cancer Survivorship,* our team reported that cancer survivors who had distressing events like Harold did showed dramatic objective and subjective changes after only three to five NET sessions. One of our study's tools for objective measurements was performing a brain scan using functional magnetic resonance imaging (fMRI) while each patient listened to a description of their distressing event. The description was based on interviews with the patient and was recorded using their own words as much as possible. We followed this same protocol before NET treatments and after NET treatments. We had a control group that went through the same protocol but did not receive any NET intervention.

The study revealed two dramatic outcomes. First, the imaging allowed us to literally see the effects of the distressing event in the patient's parahippocampus in real time before NET treatment—the parahippocampus is one of the structures in the emotional/feeling part of the brain we discussed earlier. Second, the imaging allowed us to visualize for the first time dramatic resolution of the patient's distressing event as reflected in their parahippocampus after NET treatment. Please see the brain imaging figures entitled Trauma Recovery Treatment in the color photography section for evidence of the recovery that NET can offer.

Another objective and measurable result our study revealed was the patient's nervous system's reaction to listening to the description of their distressing event. We used biofeedback equipment to measure the body's fight-or-flight response before and after NET treatments. The description of their event triggered a big fight-or-flight response before NET, but after NET their response was almost neutralized. This indicates that whenever there is a reminder of a distressing event, the fight-or-flight mechanism tends to get triggered. There is a substantial amount of independent research to corroborate this finding. This chronic triggering then cascades into another set of physiological and psychological consequences, all leading to a less happy, less healthy life.

For example, as a part of our study, repetitive disruptions were measured with assessment tools such as traumatic stress scales, mood scales, anxiety scales and quality of life scales. Many of the patients' responses registered far above the baselines. That's something to be expected, even though these patients had not said anything about psychological difficulties. What this tells us is that distressing events create a lot of traumatic stress regardless of whether the patient notices those effects. Burying it out of sight, out of mind doesn't work—just the opposite—trauma spreads its roots and grows into trees. In the language of the NET model, a distressing experience becomes a Neuro Emotional Complex (NEC), or to carry our metaphor further, a NEC grows into a patch of trees, or sometimes a forest. What surprised us about the results is how impactful even a brief NET intervention was on overall mood and psychological functions.

In looking back on your own life, what are the experiences you would prefer not to think about? Who wronged you so painfully that you get a sick feeling in your stomach when you think about them? What real or perceived failure do you not want anyone to know about because you still feel ashamed of it?

One key to resolving your NEC is to understand that it was not resolvable at the moment in time when it occurred—either there wasn't a solution then or the situation was too overwhelming for you, or both. Thus, your trauma got walled off. That's a good thing. Remember, survival is the driving force behind all of this. Sometimes you consciously block out events; for instance: *I'll deal with it in the morning after I've slept on it.*

Other times it happens subconsciously: *Let's get out of this place. It's too crowded and too expensive*—when the underlying reason you want to leave is because you somehow associate it with your ex. That same NEC might subconsciously cause you to get a new job, jump into or out of a new relationship, change your world-view, and more, all under the guise of moving on when really you're thrashing around trying to get unstuck from your ex.

There are endless ways an NEC can affect your decisions, behaviors, moods, accomplishments and sense of well-being. Yet fixing it is not an easy task. Your brain doesn't like doing this, much the same way that after a physical injury, your body doesn't like the necessary exercises for rehabilitation. And like a physical injury, an NEC often leaves scars.

You can try some NEC assessments on your own:

First, identify an experience in your life that fits the description of an NEC.

Next, rate it on a scale from zero to ten, with zero being non-stressful and ten being the highest level of distress imaginable. Go through your various experiences until you find one that you rate as being greater than six.

Identify the emotions you associate with that NEC: fear, grief, sad-ness, anger, shame or disgust. (Since, interest and joy are pleasurable emotions, usually they are not in play.) It's fine if there is only one, or more than one. It is important to actually name the emotions and write them down.

Then ask yourself, *in the context of this upsetting event, what am I saying to myself about myself?* Don't be surprised if your answers seem com-pletely illogical. They usually will. They may be harsh judgments such as *I'm a bad person . . . it's me against the world,* and so on. Go ahead and write it all down.

Once you have your emotions and self-referential statements in front of you, this allows the feeling and thinking parts of your brain to communicate with each other. Refer back to our NET study showing the parahippocampus area of the brain being highly charged before treatments. This area is where emotion-based memories are stored and where over-activation occurs when an NEC is triggered, which results in a relative disconnect from the reasoning centers in the neocortex. Getting those two parts of the brain to communicate is half the battle.

Next, close your eyes and try to focus on your emotions and self-referential statements. Then add in deep breathing while placing one of your hands flat against your forehead. Try to hold this focus for as many seconds as you can, up to one minute but not longer. You might notice an emotional release of some kind, a wave of thoughts about other related events, or maybe nothing at all. There is no right or wrong with how your brain processes these things. The goal is to bring your present-day self into the conversation while keeping aware of the emotional, illogical dialogue of the stressful event. You might also find that you think of other similar events in your life that carry the same theme, or you might have an "a-ha" moment. You might even notice some physical relaxation and hence a shift away from fight-or-flight. Any of these are healthful steps.

While this self-assessment doesn't incorporate all of the healing modalities of NET, it can be a helpful tool to combine with the other add-ons. However, some of your distressing events may be too stressful or too complex to address on your own. That's where an NET-certified practitioner utilizing the full intervention can make a big difference in your life. For more information on NET or to find a practitioner, please visit www.netmindbody.com.

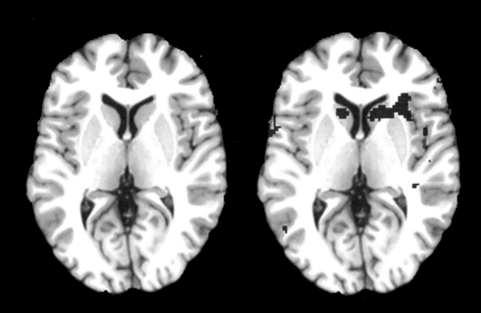

Breast Cancer Therapy. Pre-therapy (left) and post-therapy (right) functional MRI brain scan composite results show an increased activity in the basal ganglia and insula in patients with breast cancer who underwent a Health Tapestry mindfulness -based program. Greater activity in these areas reflect improvements in emotional regulation including reduced stress, anxiety and depression.

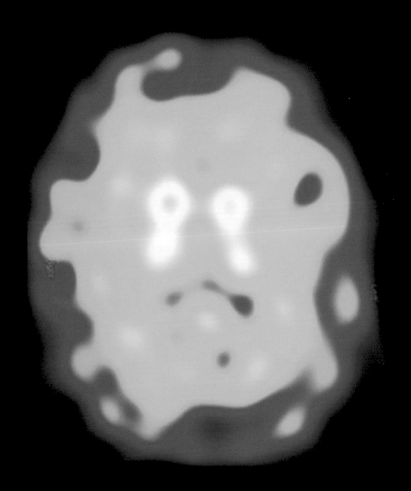

Parkinson's DiseaseTreatment. Pre-treatment (above) and post-treatment (verso) PET brain scan results for a patient with Parkinson's disease show that after three months of a Health Tapestry nutritional supplementation plan with the antioxidant N-acetyl cysteine (NAC) the patient had markedly increased dopamine levels. Dopamine is a neurotransmitter essential to clear thinking and feeling pleasure, among other functions.

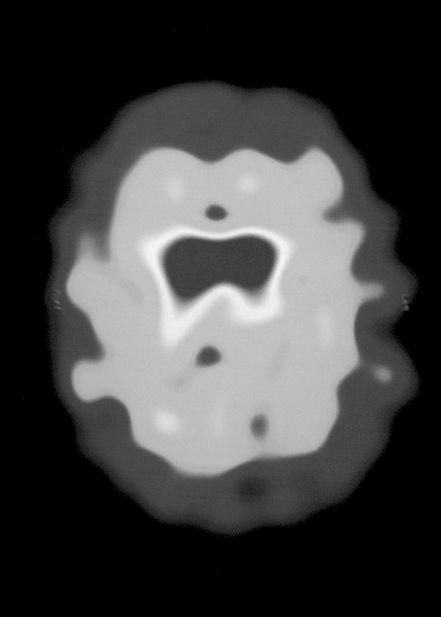

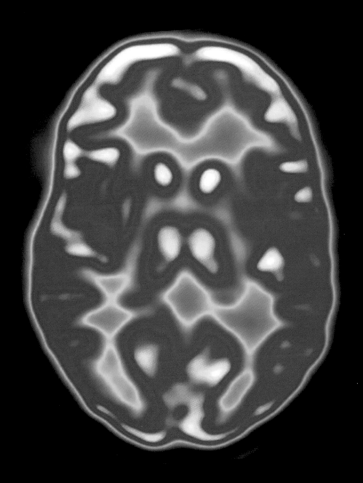

Irritable Bowel Syndrome Treatment. Pre-treatment (above) and post-treatment (verso) PET brain scan results for a patient with IBS show that after two months of Health Tapestry meal and nutritional supplementation plans the patient's overactive frontal lobes had quieted down in tandem with a lessening of their digestive disorders.

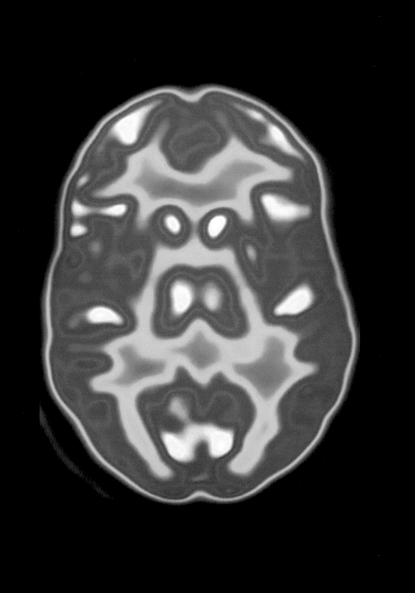

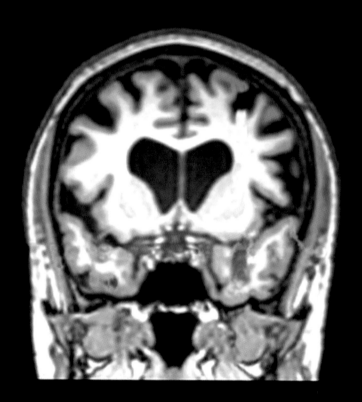

Trauma Recovery Treatment. Pre-treatment (above) and post-treatment (verso) functional MRI brain scan results for a patient with cancer-related traumatic stress show a lowering of the activation level of the parahippocampus, an area associated with emotionally stressful memories, after engaging in a Health Tapestry Neuro Emotional Technique (NET) plan for three to five sessions.

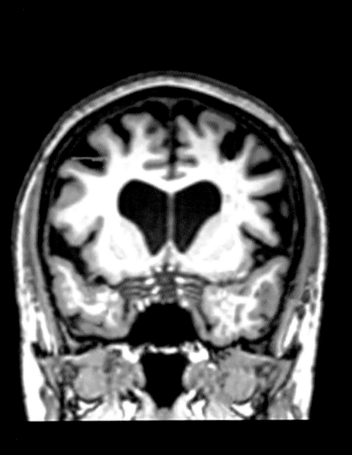

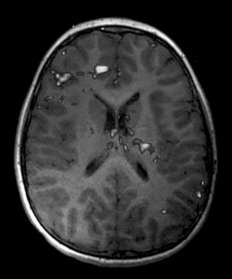 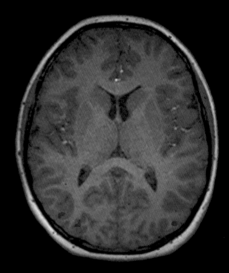

Violent Electronic Gaming Indications. Comparison of functional MRI brain scan results between an avid player of violent electronic games (left) and a nonparticipant of violent electronic games (right) show the player's increased activation in the caudate nucleus, thalamus and anterior cingulate—all areas that are part of the reward system. A growing body of research indicates there may be a cause and negative effect relationship, as well as a negative one between prolonged electronic device screen time and increased reward system activity. More research is needed.

6

WEAVING IN SLEEP HYGIENE

She was driving me crazy all night. First she's too cold, then she's too warm, then she's cold again. I kept turning the thermostat up and down. Truth is, neither one of us sleeps well these days.

—BILL, AGE 48

His snoring is so loud that I can't sleep. The whole bed vibrates from the noise! Most nights he sleeps in the den but I hate that too. I get lonely.

—CARLY, AGE 27

If you're having a difficult time getting a good night's sleep with your partner, you're not alone. Sleep problems are a common complaint among our patients. Their circumstances can be so frustrating that many couples wave the white flag and sleep in separate rooms. In fact, a survey conducted by the National Sleep Association revealed that 23 percent of married couples sleep apart.

Along with the separate-bedrooms phenomenon are more concerning findings from the Centers for Disease Control and Prevention (CDC) which show one out of three Americans don't get enough sleep. In addition, the CDC and the National Center on Sleep Disorders Research reveal an estimated 50 to 70 million American adults have sleep disorders, snoring and insomnia being among the most prevalent. Research reveals that consistently poor sleep poses serious health risks, including a greater incidence of heart disease, diabetes, weight gain and cognitive impairment. Too little sleep also increases inflammation in the body, which, as we've described, is an open invitation for illnesses. The opposite is true too—being well rested has an anti-inflammatory effect that invites good health.

It is a bit frightening when you think about the wide range of occupations of those one out of three Americans the CDC says don't get enough sleep. In a study entitled "Sleep Complaints and Fatigue of Airline Pilots" published in 2016 in the academic journal *Sleep Science*, the research found "the prevalence of sleep complaints was 34.9 percent" among the pilots in their test group. Chances are you are not a commercial pilot, but you likely are an airline passenger two or three times a year. Or, if you work as a mechanic, medical technician, first responder or in another critical position, then you can see how this can be a public safety issue. The conclusion is that getting a good night's sleep not only affects your own well-being, but also affects those depending on you. Stay-at-home parents may be too sleepy to tend to their children, teachers may be too foggy to engage their students.

Of course beds are for more than just sleeping. For those fortunate enough to be in a relationship, beds are for intimacy, late night or early morning conversations, reading or crocheting, and whatever else you and your partner enjoy. If you're not spending quality time in bed with your partner, then the rest of your relationship is likely to be cooled down, too.

One of the common goals we strive for with couples we treat is to solve their sleep problems so that they can at least be in the same bedroom, preferably in the same bed. Some of these issues can be settled simply with earplugs and nasal strips to reduce noise from snoring, adjusting the firmness of the mattress on each partner's side of the bed, turning in at the same time and agreeing on how much reading time until it's lights out, and so on.

The more complicated situations though—for both couples and singles—have responded well to the kind of integrative approach we specialize in. For instance, hormonal changes in women during menstruation, pregnancy, or menopause can drastically alter sleep patterns. Men entering midlife also typically experience hormonal changes. Even a small drop in progesterone in women and testosterone in men can disrupt their natural sleep cycles.

Other hormonal ups and downs can affect your sleep too. If you have a disagreement with your partner, family or friend, watch a scary movie before going to bed, or are traveling, it's likely your cortisol, adrenaline, melatonin and other hormonal levels will be thrown off.

Unfortunately, the pervasive anxiety that we are all perpetrators of, and victims of, isn't so easy to shut off. Your anxiety can keep you up until the wee hours of the morning as you seek comfort from late-night TV, YouTube videos of cute kittens, or romantic comedies to help mentally and physically negotiate a way to fall asleep.

Today we get about 20 percent less sleep than people did a hundred years ago. In the candlelit world of our great-grandparents, there wasn't a whole a lot to do after dark. People went to sleep earlier and were healthier for it. Many of what were once daylight activities are now "any-light" activities. Just check your Facebook, Twitter, or Instagram feed and see who is up until two in the morning and then hours later back at it at around eight. Eating dinner around six and having a bedtime snack has morphed into a nonstop eating frenzy with a late dinner followed by chips, pretzels, ice cream, popcorn, cookies and for the more serious snackers, a quick microwave of frozen pizza rolls or run to a twenty-four-hour drive-through. Aside from the calories and indigestion, eating at these late hours messes with your circadian rhythm—even after millions of years of evolution, your internal clock is still largely based on darkness and light to signal your body when it's time to sleep and when to wake up. Research findings from the National Institute on Aging Intramural Research Program, as well as other studies, report that eating late at night can override the natural "darkness means sleep" circadian prompt.

Under healthy conditions, darkness reliably sets into motion the production of melatonin by your pineal gland, a pea-sized structure embedded deep within the brain. The release of melatonin then lowers your body temperature, slows your heart rate, and makes you sleepy. Natural levels of melatonin are highest during childhood and gradually decline as we age. It's no surprise, then that at about age fifty many people begin to experience sleep disturbances. Daylight does the opposite of darkness—it inhibits the production of melatonin which then leads us to waking up. The nature of circadian prompts also helps explain why you instinctively close the drapes at night to block out bright lights.

Some prescriptions such as beta blockers for high blood pressure, NSAIDs for arthritis, and SSRIs for mood stabilization can also disrupt sleep patterns, as can over-the-counter decongestants, appetite suppressants, and more. If you suspect a prescription is interfering with your sleep, be sure to talk to your doctor, as there might be alternatives or different dosing schedules possible. But the most common sleep disrupting compound isn't at your pharmacy—no, it's at almost every busy street intersection in America: McDonald's, Dunkin' Donuts, 7-Eleven, Starbucks, Wendy's, Peet's, and thousands of other places.

We're talking about caffeine.

Everybody knows that if you drink a regular cup of coffee with its 95 mg of caffeine too close to bedtime you'll likely be in for a sleepless night. But it's not just "too close to bedtime," it's eight hours before bedtime. That's right, it takes about that long for your body to flush caffeine from your body. You may not realize that a jolt of caffeine can come from a lot of other places you otherwise don't give a second thought to. For instance, a can of Diet Coke has 46 mg of caffeine. A Hershey Scharffen Berger 82% Extra Dark Chocolate Bar has 84 mg. Even 100 percent natural Avitae bottled water has 125 mg of caffeine per bottle.

It's also important to be aware of over-the-counter medications you may take that contain caffeine or other stimulants that can interfere with sleep. For example, Excedrin Extra Strength Caplets and Tablets contain 65 mg of caffeine and Midol Menstrual Maximum Strength Caplets contain 60 mg of caffeine. Sudafed, Allegra-D and Claritin-D contain the stimulant pseudoephedrine. The "D" in the product name indicates that it contains a stimulant.

Antihistamines such as Benadryl are sometimes used as sleep aides; however we do not recommend them for that. Here's a quick biology lesson why: Histamines are good. They are natural. Your body produces them as a routine part of life and mostly maintains a balanced level all on its own. But when too much mucus forms in your nasal passages, that's a sign the histamines in your nasal lining are out of balance. Sometimes an infection or a cold are the culprits. Other times allergens and other irritants cause an unbalancing of histamine levels which then leads to excess mucous. Using antihistamines judiciously for allergic reactions is sometimes necessary. However, a few antihistamines also have a side-effect of drowsiness, and what should have been a footnote on the package has turned into a big deal through their increasing misuse as a sleep aid. In fact, you can quickly develop a tolerance for antihistamines that will interfere with your natural sleep cycle.

These medications may sedate you at first, but in time the quality of your rest will diminish. And though they might offer the illusion of an easy way out, addressing the root causes of insomnia—too much stress, too little exercise, too much sugar, too much caffeine, eating too late in the day, too much light in the bedroom from a TV or computer, an unsupportive mattress or pillow—is far more effective in the short-term and can lead to a long-term solution.

There are also some complex societal problems linked with sleeplessness. Our brains are subjected to a constant stream of information, from geopolitical threats from Russia to obsessive celebrity gossip. According to psychological studies, these preoccupations affect at least one-third of the West's population and are linked with many health issues, including insomnia. This means that our cultural over-engagement with media—24-hour cable news, junk TV, alerts and subscriptions, following every move of Beyonce and Jay Z, Kim and Kanye, *The Housewives, The Bachelor,* and other phenoms—activate our brain in ways that are often deleterious in and of themselves, but also cut into time we need for rest and relaxation. As an example of this high level of media engagement, at the time of this writing pop sensation Selena Gomez has 133 million Instagram followers. And while we love Selena and wish her every success, here's a little perspective on how large her social media fanbase is compared to other populations: Germany has a total of 80 million citizens, France has 67 million, the United Kingdom has 64 million, and Italy 62 million. Please see the brain imaging figures entitled Violent Electronic Gaming Indications in the color photography section for preliminary harmful effects from certain kinds of screen time.

Another change that can affect your sleep is the rise of home offices. One in four American households have home offices, and if your home is one of them, you can end up working way past normal quitting time, staring at a lit screen in a room with background light. For many, work doesn't ever really stop—once in bed they might still text or email from their phone. This arrangement has cast a cloud over the meaning of "after-hours." There's some satire in this. We sometimes joke with our patients who are caught up in a work-eat-sleep-repeat cycle: "It sounds like you keep banker's hours." The expression "banker's hours" has been around for several hundred years as an American colloquialism for a cushy schedule, say weekdays from 10 a.m. to 3 p.m. Then we add, "Banker's hours, like an ATM—open 24/7!"

In1964 the movie "Pajama Party," now a cult classic, was viewed by many parents, clergy and gatekeepers of morality as being quite scandalous because it dared fun-loving teens to dance along to the title track's lyrics: "Don't you know it's the latest craze, having a party wearing your PJs!" Today we joke about people who work from home and never get out of their PJs. For those who live in cramped apartments—think of the average NYC or San Francisco Bay Area 550-square-foot studio—their bed may be the only option for a workable desktop. You can imagine what an "always open for business" lifestyle does to your brain's transition, or lack thereof, to closing shop and getting some sleep. Short-changing your sleep to get ahead can instead end up putting you behind. Research shows a direct correlation between sleep deprivation among college students and their declining grade point averages.

Add to this the American misconception that sleep is no longer a necessity; it's a luxury. See for yourself: The June 2018 *Fortune* magazine article *How Sleep Became the Ultimate Luxury* addresses this. There's also the June 2018 ABC News feature *Sleep: A Necessity, Not a Luxury;* and *The Guardian's* article *How a Good Night's Sleep Became the Ultimate Status Symbol.* At the Marcus Institute, we run an Executive Health Program filled with corporate execs who live out this misconception—they are unable to sleep at night, yet some of them talk about their sleeplessness as a badge of honor as if they are contributing more to their families, careers, and communities by overworking and under-sleeping.

Data shows that insomnia is pervasive and affects a wide range of people to varying degrees based in part on their demographics. People with a college education sleep better than those without a degree; people who are employed sleep better than those who are unemployed or unable to work, and married people sleep better than those who are single. But in many of these cases, better is still not sufficient.

The conclusion is that most of us are not getting the restorative sleep we need to optimally get through the day and maintain our health. According to a recent report from the CDC, many of the problems and frustrations that have become associated with American life, including depression, anxiety, isolation, diminished libido, poor academic grades and lower work productivity can be linked to too little sleep. Indeed, the researchers believe that a person who doesn't get enough sleep is more likely to have a lower quality of life than someone who is well rested.

Healthy sleep shifts between two different cycles in a fascinating rhythm. The first shift is Non-Rem or "NREM" sleep. NREM stands for "non-rapid eye movement" activity. This is the most restful stage of sleep and includes what is referred to as "deep sleep." The other type is known as "REM" sleep. REM stands for "rapid eye movement" activity. Each type is important in its own way and serves different purposes. You typically have four to six sleep cycles per night during which you move back and forth between NREM sleep and REM sleep. Each cycle consists of 60 to 100 minutes of NREM sleep followed by a brief period of REM sleep.

Getting enough NREM sleep is particularly important for letting your body repair itself. It is during this period that tissue restores, bones and muscles grow, and the immune system revitalizes. REM sleep is particularly important for heightening cognitive abilities such as those associated with learning and memory, as well as for regulating neurotransmitters that affect mood stability.

There are many more revelations about the value of sleep. It is important to note that up until about 20 years ago, there wasn't a lot of vigorous scientific discussion about this because it was thought that the body would adapt to just about any amount of sleep. We are adaptive animals after all. For instance, over time the brain can sublimate a continually disruptive noise into a barely noticeable background sound. As a result, the thunderous clanking and screeching of the Q train as it passes through Brooklyn all day hardly registers with longtime residents of Brighton Beach.

Or take people who are born into or move to cold or hot weather regions. Their bodies acclimate to their environment. For example, when asked about what kind of weather he'd wear short sleeves in, one New Englander answered, "I'm good down to about 50 degrees in short sleeves and shorts and sandals. I also assume that I'll put my hands in my pockets." Tell that to this woman from the Southwest: "I live in Arizona and will wear long sleeves for work on days that reach 115 plus. I normally won't wear short sleeves in temperatures lower than 85."

This adaptive quality, as it was applied to earlier sleep theories, suggested that if you got only five hours of sleep your body would adjust. If you got four hours your body would adjust. You can imagine the excitement over this way of thinking. Get more done and enjoy more of life instead of "wasting" time sleeping.

But then researchers began saying, "Wait a minute." As it turned out, it wasn't an even swap between time asleep and time awake. In the 1990s evidence began to emerge about cognitive deficiencies from not getting enough rest. Later, other health risks emerged as a result of sleep deprivation. And today it is widely supported by volumes of studies that sleep is vitally important to your entire body-mind ecosystem.

Sleep turns out to be a matter of life and death for those serving in the military. In a report from the Walter Reed Army Institute of Research, the findings include the following summation: "Sleep is a biological need, critical for sustaining the mental abilities needed for success on the battlefield. Soldiers require seven to eight hours of good quality sleep every 24-hour period to sustain operational readiness. Soldiers who lose sleep will accumulate a sleep debt over time that will seriously impair their performance. The only way to pay off this debt is by obtaining the needed sleep. The demanding nature of military operations often creates situations where obtaining sleep may be difficult or even impossible for more than short periods. While essential for many aspects of operational success, sheer determination or willpower cannot offset the mounting effects of inadequate sleep.

"Therefore, sleep should be viewed as being as critical as any logistical item of resupply, like water, food, fuel and ammunition. Commanders need to plan proactively for the allocation of adequate sleep for themselves and their subordinates."

Is sleep any less critical for you and your loved ones? If sleep is necessary for war, then certainly it is necessary for peace, too.

We now have an even wider understanding of the purpose of a good night's rest. When you sleep, your metabolism slows. Your heart rate drops and so does your blood pressure. Your level of human growth hormone rises, which stimulates the repair of old cells and the production of new ones. (Exercise is another way to boost human growth hormone.) Sleep is a period during which your body reverses the clock—it de-ages. Missed sleep is a missed opportunity for youthfulness. In fact, hormone levels of the sleep deprived are similar to those of much older people.

Sleep is also a way of dealing with stress. Despite many other biological functions tapering off during sleep, your brain remains surprisingly active. For instance, there are early indications from ongoing research to suggest that while sleeping, you sort through events of the day, processing information and even solving problems, and that your neurotransmitters—the brain's important natural chemicals that help you think, learn and regulate your mood—reset to their normal daily levels. In contrast, when you don't get enough sleep your neurotransmitters go haywire; for instance the neurotransmitter glutamate rises which makes your body pump out more of the stress hormone cortisol which in turn can result in weight gain, spikes in blood sugar and difficulties in paying attention.

The sleep-weight connection is intriguing too. Studies show that people who routinely don't get enough sleep are at greater risk for obesity. Scientists think this is because a lack of sleep reduces the production of the metabolic hormones that regulate your appetite. This can be a real Rubik's Cube. How do you keep from eating when your appetite is roaming free and you're too tired to corral it back in? That's why we advise: when you feel hungry at night just GO TO BED.

7

HEALTH TAPESTRY SLEEP PLAN

Everyone has an occasional bout with insomnia. The most common form is known as transient insomnia. It only lasts for a few nights and is typically caused by a temporary event like jet lag, excitement, illness, or a change in schedule. It often resolves itself.

The next level up is called short-term insomnia. It lasts up to three weeks, and is often caused by life-altering events like the death of a loved one, job change, divorce, or prolonged worries. It can potentially resolve itself, but it's pretty ordinary to have some kind of intervention. As is true with many health conditions, short-term problems can turn into long-term ones if they aren't resolved sooner rather than later.

Insomnia, just as a stand-alone word or with the qualifiers "persistent" or "chronic," refers to sleeplessness that persists for more than a month. It occurs as a symptom of an underlying medical condition like chronic pain, reflux, clinical depression and anxiety disorder.

Remedies depend on each person's situation, though there are some general guidelines that work across the board. For example, exercise and mild stretching can relieve symptoms of restless leg syndrome (RLS). This condition is characterized by a tingling feeling, and in some cases pain, along with an uncomfortable urge to move your legs; it usually worsens when you lie down. The cause is unknown, although it is often associated with other medical problems such as peripheral neuropathy, diabetes mellitus, anemia or rheumatoid arthritis. There are also some medications that can help with RLS. It is important to consult with your doctor about treatment for the underlying issues.

Teeth grinding—bruxism—is another common problem that can keep you up at night, not to mention damage your teeth and gums. In severe cases, bruxism can cause headaches and neck and jaw problems. The main treatment is to wear a mouth guard at night that will hold your bite in place and prevent grinding. We recommend a custom molded one from your dentist rather than the generic over-the-counter type. Bruxism is most often an indicator of unmanaged stress, so it is important to address not only the physical symptoms but also the emotions driving you to grind your teeth. Often you won't even know you are doing it, but your dentist will be able to tell almost immediately. This is one of many reasons why it's important to have regular dental checkups. Other reasons are that plaque buildup, tooth decay, periodontal disease and other dental issues can be indicators of some hidden heath conditions.

Working late can also keep you from getting a good night's rest. We understand that sometimes things get pushed to the last minute. Maybe you need to respond right away to a time-sensitive email or set up your Powerpoint presentation for an early morning meeting. The important thing is that you create a curfew and stick to it. Habitually working late without a clear quitting time chips away at the important function your personal life is meant to fulfill.

It helps to make your home workspace a separate area from the part you relax in. If your workspace is also where you relax, then for at least two hours before you go to sleep put away your laptop and stop reading anything work-related. Dim the lights or have a reading light for that novel you're into, listen to your favorite music, or do whatever else soothes you. If you like to watch TV, avoid shows that are too violent or too suspenseful—they can jack up your senses when you need to calm them down so you can sleep.

As we mentioned earlier, caffeine consumption calls for some extra planning because it takes about eight hours to get cleared from your system. This means that if 10:00 o'clock is usually lights out—we recommend 10:00 for just about everyone—set 2:00 in the afternoon as your cutoff for any caffeine, including hidden sources like soft drinks, chocolate and over-the-counter medications.

Some of these medications may have natural alternatives. For example, drink water for a headache or take calcium for leg cramps. When you have congestion and excess mucous, try an old-fashioned hot steam with eucalyptus. Fill a pot with water and bring it to a boil. Put in some eucalyptus leaves and let it sit for a minute or two. Carefully remove the pot from the stove and place it safely on a table. Then put a towel over your head and the pot to make a type of enclosed tent, or leave it open-aired and ventilated if you prefer, and inhale the vapors for about five minutes.

According to the National Sleep Foundation, snoring is probably the most common of all sleep problems, affecting about 90 million Americans each year. Though we tend to think of snoring as a male issue, women are right up there: about four out of 10 men snore compared to three out of 10 women—and another strike against antihistamines is that they exacerbate snoring.

At one time or another you probably have, or will, elbow your partner in the middle of the night to get him or her to turn on their side or to at least quiet down. If that doesn't work, and neither does anything else you can think of, the two of you might find yourself in separate bedrooms, which, as we discussed, can lead to a strain on your physical and emotional intimacy.

You might be asking yourself *how is it possible that I breathe normally and quietly during the day but at night I snore as loud as a train?* The answer is that when you sleep the muscles in your throat relax causing the airway passage that brings oxygen to and from your lungs to narrow. The fluttering sound is created by the vibrations of these relaxed parts rubbing against each other.

There are other factors that figure in, too. If you have a cold or seasonal allergies you're more likely to snore. If you are overweight or past midlife you're more likely to snore. If you eat dairy products or don't exercise you are also more likely to snore.

Severe snoring, though, is in a category of its own and is usually the result of a condition called sleep apnea. That's when your breathing is actually interrupted, sometimes hundreds of times a night. Sleep apnea requires medical attention. The word "apnea" is Greek in origin and translates to English as "without breath," which aptly describes this potentially life-threatening condition. About four percent of men and two percent of women have sleep apnea. The sound of your partner gasping for breath can be extremely distressing. Very often though you are the first one to become aware of your partner's condition and the first to urge them to seek medical care.

If your snoring is not severe, there are a number of steps you can take for some relief:

Lose Weight. If you are overweight, especially if you have a double chin, losing weight can help reduce or even eliminate snoring. Here's a reference point: if you lose 10 pounds, you will shrink your neck size by about one inch. The loss of just a few pounds can make a real difference in your breathing and snoring. Our Health Tapestry Weight Loss Plan is a good place to start.

Skip the Nightcap. Alcohol relaxes your muscles, including your throat muscles, so if you are tempted to drink before bedtime, don't. If you are an average non-snorer, drinking even a minimal amount of alcohol before bed is likely to make you snore as much as a habitual snorer would. A habitual snorer who drinks alcohol before bed is at greater risk of developing sleep apnea.

Stop Smoking. The more you smoke, the more you snore. Smoking, or even regular exposure to second-hand smoke, irritates your throat and causes congestion in your nasal passages and lungs. A tobacco habit can cause inflammation of the tissues lining your airways, narrowing the passage even further. Plus, nicotine is a stimulant, which is the last thing you want when you're ready to fall sleep, and research shows that you'll more likely wake up grumpier than a nonsmoker. If you need help quitting, we recommend the smoking cessation program developed at Duke University or the JeffQuit program we developed at the Marcus Institute.

Sleep on Your Side. Sleeping on your side can minimize the effect of your relaxed throat muscles and airway passages. There are special pillows designed for this. Or you can try this do-it-yourself hack with a tennis ball: Sew a sock to the back of your pajama top and put a tennis ball in the sock. When you're sleeping, if you try to lie on your back the ball will sharply remind you to do otherwise. Soon enough you will get used to sleeping on your side and that tennis ball can have a second life as a toy for your dog to play with.

Sleep on a Firm Pillow. A firm pillow supports your head at an angle that positions your tongue and jaw to rest forward, which in turn helps your throat and airways stay open.

Elevate Your Bed. Adjustable beds are more common than ever. However, if you don't have one, there is an easy fix: Place a foam wedge or rolled-up towels under your mattress to get about a four-inch lift. This elevated position can make breathing easier and keep your tongue and jaw resting forward.

Eat Light at Night. Late-night eating invites snoring because the process of digestion also relaxes your throat and tongue muscles. But if you must eat at late hours—by "must" we mean your work schedule or other responsibilities have pushed you to an odd hour (not must as in "I'm craving cinnamon rolls"), avoid dairy products because they cause sinus mucous; avoiding dairy is something we recommend whether you snore or not. Make your dish as light as possible, which means minimal fat, even the good kind. A smoothie or chopped salad with a touch of extra-virgin olive oil and lemon is good, or if you want something warm, steamed brown rice or another grain is fine.

Snacks before bed fall into a gray area. If you've had a full dinner but still have the munchies, you might want to try drinking a glass of cold water. Sometimes your body's messages can seem confusing: for instance, you might be thirsty and/or tired but interpret the signals as hunger. If you still want a little something, have a couple of spoonfuls of non-dairy soy or rice frozen dessert; just remember to keep the grams of sugar per serving in the single digits. Or have a glass of unsweetened non-dairy flax, soy, rice or almond milk. We like flax milk because it's the only one of these that contains the heart-healthy omega-3s, plus it has a nice flavor.

Exercise. Exercising will tone your whole body including those parts involved in reducing or eliminating snoring. This includes aerobic exercises that strengthen your upper airways. One caveat—do your workout at least three hours before bedtime. Exercising any later than that could keep you up.

Other natural remedies that can help reduce snoring include gargling with diluted peppermint oil, taking a hot shower using eucalyptus aromatherapy to open your airways, and doing yoga. These poses in particular may help: Kapalbhati, which concentrates on sinuses; Bhastrika, which centers on inhalations and exhalations being of equal durations; and Nadi Shodhana, which emphasizes nostril breathing. Most meditative practices, including mindfulness, which we recommend for everyone, focus on breathing. The more easefully we breathe, the better.

Some over-the-counter products can be temporarily helpful. These include sprays to moisten your nasal passages, sprays to lubricate and tone your throat muscles, and chin strips to position your tongue and jaw in a way that keeps your airways open. They don't work for everyone, but they work for enough people that it may be worth giving them a try. Please consult with your doctor or pharmacist for their recommendations.

Structural abnormalities that cause snoring such as a deviated septum, nasal polyps, enlarged adenoids or tonsils, or a long uvula or soft palate are best evaluated by an ear, nose and throat (ENT) specialist. Your dentist can also tell you about several effective orthodontic appliances to reposition your tongue and jaw and open up your airways—some are worn inside the mouth, and some are fitted around the head and chin to position the lower jaw.

Depending on your condition, your doctor may recommend that you see a sleep specialist who might advise you to spend a night at a sleep clinic, where your sleep patterns can be observed. In some cases, a throat or nose corrective procedure may be advisable. For instance, in snoreplasty, a scarring agent is injected into soft tissue to stiffen the palate and thereby improve your airflow. Somnoplasty is a procedure in which a heated, thin needle is inserted into excess throat tissue to open up your airway. Uvulopalatopharyngoplasty (UPPP), the most aggressive of these kinds of treatments, is the surgical removal of excess throat tissue.

Aside from just fixing a snoring problem, the first and most important remedy to start with is to commit to making sleeping well a priority in your life. This is often referred to as good sleep hygiene.

Your bedtime routines are an important part of good sleep hygiene. For instance, your routine might be to have a piece of fruit or a small snack and then brush your teeth before turning in. Or maybe you watch the opening monologue by Colbert, Kimmel, or Fallon and then call it quits. Or you decide what you're going to wear the next day, brush your hair, read a book. These predictable patterns send signals to your body that sleep is soon to come. They cue your body to start the process of falling asleep before you even get into bed. Your body becomes conditioned to these routines, so if you're on and off with your late night TV laughs or reading, you send a mixed message: "It might be time to sleep or there might be something else coming up."

A similar principle applies to keeping a consistent bedtime. If you go to bed regularly at ten o'clock, your biorhythms are already anticipating sleep hours before then. If you have staggered bedtimes, for instance, one night you're in by eleven, the next at one in the morning, then to make up for that the next night you're in early at nine, and you keep doing this, your internal clock doesn't know what time it is.

We also suggest getting into bed a bit before you want to fall asleep. That way you can settle in, get comfortable, have an intimate exchange if you are sleeping with someone, and maybe even get a few extra minutes of bonus sleep. If it's been a rough day, you might want to do some quiet meditation or stress reduction exercises. This time is yours. It's best for couples to try to go to bed at the same time and adhere to the same sleep schedule, even if one of you has to get up earlier than the other. Staying on the same schedule is not only important for intimacy, but also for restful sleep for both of you.

Another aspect of your sleep hygiene is thinking of your bedroom as a sanctuary. In that way it becomes a place where you can enjoy serenity—fresh flowers or scented candles can add ambience as well. This is an important contrast to a bedroom you associate with as a place to pay bills, stash papers, store old computers, or play on your phone.

And never mind that your mother told you to make your bed every day, we tell you the same thing. Even if you don't get around to it until just before bedtime, do it. That way, your bed will feel neat and inviting and not a reminder of the day's loose ends. Splurging on the best sheets that you can afford with the highest thread count possible is another way to make your sleep more soothing. When you wake up, if you feel back or neck pain, your mattress or pillow may not be giving you proper support. In that case, it may be time to purchase a new mattress. A good one is well worth the investment. Also, switch out your pillow if it's old, even if it's still comfortable. Over time, pillows gather dust mites, allergens and other irritants which can contribute to congestion, snoring and restlessness. Consider a new pillow to be an annual investment.

If you want more help with your sleep hygiene, a magnesium and calcium supplement taken as needed at bedtime will have a calming effect on your body. We advise a 1,000 mg calcium/500 mg magnesium combination. Another natural sedative you can try is the amino acid tryptophan. Tryptophan is the compound found in turkey, which is one reason why you might find yourself feeling sleepy after a turkey dinner. A usual dosage is a 500 mg tryptophan capsule supplement at bedtime.

The natural hormone melatonin, when taken as a supplement, is also effective for bringing on sleep. We recommend taking one to six mg at bedtime. We base these dosages on our clinical experience and numerous studies on melatonin and sleep. A potential downside to taking it at the higher dosage is you may find you are still sleepy in the morning and well into the day. However, it doesn't work for some people unless they take a high dose. You can try it and see how it works for you.

Aside from the commonly known natural herbal remedy of sipping a cup of hot chamomile tea before turning in, there are several other "sleep" herbs you can explore in combination formulas. Soothing herbal teas often include passion flower, valerian, hops, skull cap, and gotu kola along with flavorful lemon, apple, orange, ginger and licorice.

The safe use of herbal medicines goes back for thousands of years; the earliest known usage dating to 5,000 years ago in China. The ancient Greeks and Romans also used herbs for healing as did Native American Indians. Yet, it is important to be mindful of how these powerful natural herbal compounds interact with modern pharmaceuticals. Some research shows that certain herbs can be counteractive to particular medications. For example, if you are taking sedatives like Klonopin or Ambien, talk with your doctor first before adding any herbal sleep aids like passion flower.

We do prescribe sleep medications from time to time because, in some cases, simply getting back on track is the most immediate concern. We take this approach with reluctance; it's a one-time prescription for no more than three weeks, and with careful monitoring because of potentially significant tolerance build-ups, drug interactions and side effects. You can also download an app with background white noise or soft music to help you sleep.

8

WEAVING IN EXERCISE

Diet, genetics, attitude and exercise are among the most common factors associated with good health. Okay, so you decide to switch from soda to green tea and from Thousand Island dressing to oil and lemon. Those are good starts for meal planning. You know that heart disease runs in your family so you decide to get regular checkups for your blood pressure and cholesterol. And you've had enough stressful situations in your life so you make a new rule: "I'm going to breathe through the rough moments and difficult people I encounter every day, being as mindful as possible." All of these are good moves. If you are like most people, it's an ongoing process to consistently get to a place with more balance.

But exercise? Odds are you haven't made a dent in that one, and you're not alone. According to a study published in June of 2018 by the CDC, only 23 percent of Americans get enough exercise—and the bar is pretty low: just 20 minutes a day of moderate exercise is the CDC's recommendation. If you park your car at the back of the parking lot and walk from there to the store, take the stairs instead of the elevator, wash your car, rake leaves, garden, or any combination of these and other easy efforts, you will get in your recommended 20 minutes a day.

A good start would be to add in about 10 minutes twice a week for strength training. Start by using two 3- to 5-pound dumbbells for three sets of 10 to 12 repetitions each for arm curls, overhead lifts, lunges and squats.

You don't need to purchase anything to get started. You don't need a gym. You don't need a personal trainer. You don't need a Beachbody 21 Day Fix or Insanity

Workout video, or a *Dancing With the Stars* or *The Biggest Loser* workout—of course if any of these things help you then definitely follow their lead. Or they might be things you want to add to your routine once you get started. We want you to know that there is no mystery to integrating exercise into your lifestyle. We want you to get in the habit of following a routine without giving a second thought to its necessity and its rewards, just like you do with having clean socks to wear every day.

If you want to pursue a bikini body or six-pack abs, go ahead. But let's be honest, most of us aren't going to make it to that level, nor do we need to. A better focus is on increasing cardiovascular tone, flexibility, balancing major muscle groups, maximizing function and strengthening your core as elements of peak conditioning. Start by getting off the couch and increasing your activity level by 20 minutes a day. If you are already doing this, then add another 20 minutes. Exercise is like eating green vegetables—most of us don't have to worry about getting too much.

We emphasize that fitness is often as much a psychological challenge as a physical one. Approximately three-quarters of all American adults are overweight or obese—we all want to feel like we belong, but you don't want to be a member of this three-quarters club. It will be better to assert your individuality and be with the one-quarter that stays more fit and trim. We know how difficult peer and family pressure can be if you want to stake your claim. We face it too. At times our friends have said to both of us things like:

"Enough with the rabbit food! Have some fun!"

"You make me feel guilty watching you exercise."

"I feel fat standing next to you."

But the simple truth is the more you take care of yourself, the more you can give to those you love. Sometimes doing what's right means going your own way, and maybe, just maybe, those you are closest to will be inspired to follow your example.

If you are over fifty, being fit and trim likely will mean you need to be a lot more creative than when you were younger. In those earlier days you could go running or meet up with friends for an afternoon of basketball. But as you age, your joints can't take the shock of high-impact sports, and even relatively minor injuries such as pulled muscles often take longer to heal. That's when reinventing your exercise program needs to kick in. For example, you can shoot hoops with your friends but not play the kind of game that leads to contact driving through the lane. You can swim at a leisurely pace if you like the water, or ride an elliptical if you like the motion. The point is, just because you have gotten older and can't do high intensity sports anymore doesn't mean you can't adapt to very enjoyable and fulfilling modifications.

In fact, studies show that inactivity breeds more inactivity. It's pretty much a downward slide unless some kind of intervention puts the breaks on. Wherever it is you are, on a slope or flat ground, we encourage you to become more mindful of your daily physical activity. Whatever your baseline is, you can increase it starting today. There are a lot of things you can choose that count toward increased activity even if you don't think of them as exercise in a traditional sense. For example, getting down on the floor with your children or grandchildren and lovingly lifting them and twirling their little bodies, playing tug of war with your dog to see who gets the squeeze toy, or scrubbing the tub and vacuuming all count toward physical activity. You may like or need to do them anyway, so it's a real bonus that they count. From there, add some planned physical activities—the more physically active you are, the more you can literally create a healthier you; the less physically active, the less of a healthier you.

EXERCISE IMPROVES BRAIN FUNCTION

There's another aspect to exercise that comes up in many conversations with our patients. They ask, "Will this help me think better?" It's common knowledge that doing crossword puzzles and games like sudoku can help keep you mentally sharp, but now there is definitive evidence that physical exercise is even more effective for building cognitive health than those brain exercises are. Studies reveal that depression, anxiety, memory loss, dementia, diminished reaction time, and more can be abated by physical exercise. When you exercise, neurotransmitters are released that improve brain function and slow down natural aging declines in cognition. A resulting decrease in inflammation is another one of the mechanisms believed to contribute to these qualities.

Another positive effect of exercise is something you may have heard referred to as "runner's high." This is when endorphins released by the brain lead to a sense of overall well-being, which some runners even describe as euphoria. These endorphins, as well as related serotonin and norepinephrine, can also be released through mild forms of physical activity like walking on a nature trail or mowing the lawn. Physical activity at virtually any level improves the quality of your life, including helping you cope with stress. If you are not exercising now, then you are less adept at coping, and more likely to feel tied in knots. As you begin to put your Health Tapestry Plan together, you will see that physical activity is as integral to your health as nutrition, temperament, sleep, and more, and impacts the way you live every day—cognitively, physically and emotionally. Specifically, studies show regular physical activity can:

- Improve immune functioning so your body can resist disease
- Help you sleep better so you feel energized
- Reduce the risk of breast, prostate and other cancers
- Decrease inflammation so you have less illness
- Keep your muscles and joints strong to help you stay injury-free and pain-free
- Promote good digestion and regularity
- Increase blood flow and vitality

We've discussed all of the logical reasons why exercise is invaluable. Now let's move on to some reasons beyond data points and risk rates. The primary one is that exercising can be fun. No doubt you understand the fun part of going for a bike ride.

Exercise can also be an immersive experience. The immersion part involves tapping into your self-awareness about how your body responds to exercise, the good and the bad. For instance, that old adage "No pain, no gain" can put you at risk for serious injury. Sure, testing your limits is healthy, but at a certain point, no means no. Better to stay attuned to what your body is telling you than to do some kind of mental jiujitsu to show how tough you are.

Yoga is an excellent example of your body, mind and spirit being engaged for well-being. But not everyone wants to be a yogi. Some people find working out at the gym provides a profound sense of well-being while others find being outdoors gives them that sense of emotional restoration, mental clarity and spiritual tranquility. The main takeaway is the intrinsic value of exercise is far greater than just physical.

If you have a romantic partner, regular and consistent exercise can add more spark to your relationship. Here are just a few of the many benefits to partnering up:

If you've both agreed to a workout date, then you two are less likely to come up with excuses for why you can't make it.

Working out together can help you two get back in sync physically, emotionally, mentally and spiritually.

Doing physical activity side by side opens a bit of peeking (please no gawking!) at one another's bodies that can lead to more intimacy between you two.

Numerous studies show that fit people are more likely to feel desirable, and as a result have more physical intimacy than less-fit people. This is as true for college students as it is for people old enough to be their parents and grandparents. For example, a 2000 study conducted at Harvard University with 160 male and female swimmers in their 40s and 60s linked regular physical activity with more frequent and enjoyable encounters.

Sometimes it can be difficult to schedule exercise dates with your partner. If this becomes an ongoing issue, just work out on your own. Or consider setting up a home-based fitness plan that might make it easier for you to exercise together.

The goal is to do some kind of physical activity together. If it's you on the tread-mill and your partner on the StairMaster, that's fine. If it's you shoveling snow off the sidewalk and your partner chipping ice off the car windshield, that's okay. If it's late and you two can only squeeze in a walk around the neighborhood, that's good enough.

Setting up your own home-based fitness program for yourself usually doesn't require much of an investment, especially if you enjoy walking, hiking, gardening and other outdoor activities. If you want to spring for equipment, we suggest an elliptical machine, exercise bike, stair stepper, rowing machine, or treadmill.

When it comes to home-based strength training, we recommend investing in a couple of 3-, 5-, 10- or 12-pound dumbbells, an exercise ball, a set of exercise resistance bands, and an exercise mat. An exercise bench is not essential.

DIVING IN

Okay, you've got the mojo and the equipment, now it's time to get exercising.

If you are able and willing to begin a full workout now, our recommended 30-Minute Three-Step Health Tapestry Exercise Plan opens with stretching, moves on to strength training and ends with core strengthening. This program is best when done three days a week. However, if you can't make that commitment, start with stretching or the core exercises and then build up from there when you are ready.

First, be aware of keeping good posture, breathing comfortably, moving slowly and maintaining overall good form in stretching, strength training, walk-ing, swimming, yoga, you name it. That's not so you'll look good during your workout—though you will—it's to help you get the most from your routine and avoid injuries.

Those are the basics, but we all know some rules are meant to be broken. For instance, though getting a full-body workout by emphasizing all major muscle groups is the ideal, it's okay to modify that if you want to spend more time on conditioning a particular area. For example, if you are a man you might want to focus more on fat build-up around your midsection and if you are a woman on your hips.

30-MINUTE THREE-STEP HEALTH TAPESTRY EXERCISE PLAN

STEP ONE: 10 MINUTES

Stretching

The loss of flexibility that tends to occur with aging makes stretching an essential element of your everyday fitness. Flexibility helps keep you agile and prevent injuries. In addition, stretching can help counteract those sedentary hours stuck behind a desk or glued to a computer. The beginner-level stretches described below offer a path to a healthier, better-feeling you.

Hamstring Stretch

Your hamstrings are the muscles on the back of your legs that support your thighs and derriere. If you don't have a lot of physical activity, your hams will stiffen up and often trigger lower back pain.

- Sit in a chair or on the side of your bed with your feet flat on the floor.

- Slide your left leg out straight in front of you, keeping your left heel on the floor and toes pointing up. Your right foot still remains flat on the floor in its original position.

- Keeping your back straight, slowly lean your chest forward bending only at your waist until you feel a gradual pull on the back of your left thigh. Hold your body in this tilted position with your head up, stomach in, and shoulders back.

- Hold this stretch for 20 seconds.

- Repeat three times with a five-second rest between stretches.

- Then switch to your right leg and follow the same steps.

You can also do this stretch with a partner. In that case you are doing what is referred to as a "passive" stretch; that is, you allow your partner to control your movement into a comfortable position. It's important that you communicate with your partner when you feel any pain so they can ease up.

- Lie on your back with your legs extended while your partner faces your feet within hands reach.

- Your partner lifts your left leg (your right leg remains extended in its original position) by putting one hand on your heel and one hand on your thigh. They then gently raise your leg. Bend your leg slightly at the knee so that you don't hyperextend your hamstring.

- Then switch to your right leg and follow the same steps.

Pectoral Stretch

Your "pecs" are your chest muscles. This exercise also helps stretch your arms and shoulders.

- Stand in a doorway with your feet shoulder-width apart.

- Place your left arm against the frame at a 90-degree angle and place your right elbow against the door frame.

- Step forward with your left foot until you feel a mild stretch in your chest area.

- Hold for this stretch for 20 seconds.

- Repeat three times with a five-second rest between stretches.

- Then switch to your right arm against the frame at a 90-degree angle and place your left elbow against the door frame, step forward with your right foot, and follow the same steps.

To do this stretch with a partner, sit on the floor with your legs crossed and your hands behind your head. Your partner squats behind you, facing your back. Your partner then places their knee in between your shoulder blades and slowly pulls back on your elbows until you feel a comfortable stretch. It's important that you communicate with your partner when you feel any pain so they can ease up.

Latissimus "Lat" Stretch

Your "lats" are your upper back muscles. This exercise requires an exercise ball and is best done with a partner.

- Kneel down behind the ball. Position both of your hands on top of the ball vertically on their sides with palms facing each other (like parallel karate chops), distanced apart equal to the ball's diameter.

- Slowly lower your chest, leaning on the ball and rolling it away from your body while straightening your arms until you feel a stretch in your armpits. Roll the ball to manipulate the stretch while your partner stands in front of the ball to help stabilize it.

- Hold this stretch for 20 seconds.

- Repeat three times with a five-second rest between stretches.

Calf Stretch

This is a classic stretch. It's especially helpful for women who wear high heels and find that their legs hurt at the end of the day, but it's equally important for men, too.

- Stand at the bottom of a staircase and hold on to the railing with both hands.

- Move the balls of your feet onto the first step, leaving your heels dangling.

- Slowly lower your heels until you feel a tight stretch behind your shin.

To do this with a partner, lay flat on your back with your partner at your feet. Your partner then takes your left foot in their hand, and presses your heel up against their chest until you feel a comfortable stretch. Then switch to your right foot and follow the same steps. It's important that you communicate with your partner when you feel any pain so they can ease up.

- Hold this stretch for 20 seconds.

- Repeat three times with a five-second rest between stretches.

Three Gentle and Quick Stretches for When You Are On the Go
Relax Your Lower Back

Stand up tall, with your feet shoulder-width apart and your hands clasped behind your back. Pull back with your hands until you feel a comfortable stretch in your lower back. Hold this stretch for 10 seconds. Repeat three times with a five-second rest between stretches.

Stretch Your Shoulders and Upper Back

Stand up tall, with your feet shoulder-width apart and your hands at your side. Reach your arms over your head, breath in, and gently curve your upper torso backward until you feel a comfortable stretch. Hold this stretch for 10 seconds. Repeat three times with a five-second rest between stretches.

Loosen Your Hips

Stand up tall, with your feet about two feet apart. While keeping your stomach in and your pelvis tilted forward, keep widening your stance until you feel a comfortable stretch in your derriere, hips and upper thighs. Hold this stretch for 10 seconds. Repeat three times with a five-second rest between stretches.

STEP TWO: 10 MINUTES
STRENGTH TRAINING

Musculoskeletal strength training is important for both women and men. It helps build bone density, enhance muscle mass, improve mood, and more. Some fear that strength training will add bulkiness, but that is almost never the case if done according to the Health Tapestry Exercise Plan. The goal isn't muscle bulk but improved muscle function, tone, stability and resilience. Diminished muscle capacity is a normal part of the aging process and strength training is one of the best tools for keeping your body more youthful and vibrant.

Weights are most commonly used for strength training. Resistance bands are just as effective. We recommend a few general guidelines:

- Do three sets of 10 to 12 repetitions (reps) for each exercise.

- For each repetition, count *1, 2* on the exertion, and *1, 2, 3* on the release. Take little or no rest between reps.

- Rest for 30 seconds between sets.

- In between different exercises, allow yourself a 30- to 60-second break. These breaks may push your workout into the "Goldilocks Zone," which is the place right in between too little exercise and too much exercise for optimal health effects.

SHOULDERS

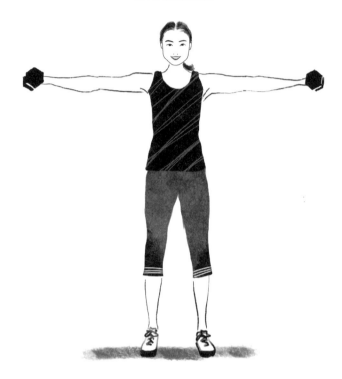

* *Warm-up for weightlifting: first do one set of 5 to 10 repetitions without weights.*

- Stand tall with your feet shoulder-width apart and your knees slightly bent.

- Hold a 3- to 5-pound weight in each hand with your arms stretching downward at your sides, and palms facing inward.

- Slightly bend your elbows and slowly lift your arms out sideways to bring the weights to shoulder level, being careful not to lift your arms higher than your shoulders.

- Lower the weights back to the starting position.

- Do three sets of 10 to 12 repetitions. Take little or no rest between reps.

- Rest for 30 seconds between sets.

- Variation: Instead of slowly lifting your arms out sideways, slowly lift them straight out in front of you, or alternate slowly lifting one arm at a time.

CHEST

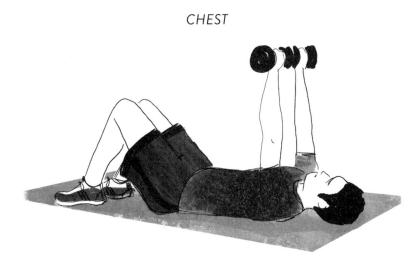

* Warm-up for weightlifting: first do one set of five to 10 repetitions without weights.

- Lie on your back on a mat or heavy towel.

- Hold ten-pound weights in each hand, palms facing downward, arms straight beside you.

- Slowly bend your forearms upward until your elbows are bent and the weights are at chest level.

- Slowly straighten your arms upward until the weights are extended above your chest. The weights will tend to move close together with your upward motion, so try to keep them the same distance apart as when you started at chest level.

- Slowly lower the weights back to the chest-level starting position.

- Do three sets of 10 to 12 repetitions. Take little or no rest between reps.

- Rest for 30 seconds between sets.

BICEPS

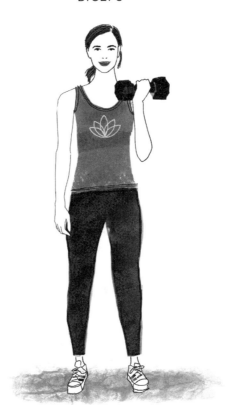

- * *Warm-up for weightlifting: first do one set of five to 10 repetitions without weights.*

- Stand with your feet shoulder-width apart, and pick up a weight in your right hand.

- Place your arms at your side, palms facing up, with your elbows close to your sides.

- Curl your right arm until your elbows bend past 90 degrees.

- Lower to the starting position.

- Do three sets of 10 to 12 repetitions. Take little or no rest between reps.

- Rest for 30 seconds between sets.

- Switch arms and follow the same steps.

TRICEPS

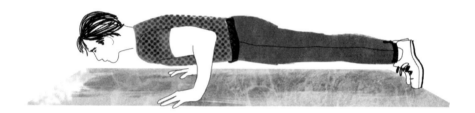

- This is a variation on the military-style push-up. Get on your hands and knees on a mat or heavy towel. Place your palms flat on the floor as you would for a standard push-up–shoulder-width apart, wrists under shoulders, and your arms extended straight but not too straight so that your elbows don't lock. Keep your neck and head aligned with your spine in a plank-like position. Hold your stomach in tight to support your back.

- Lower yourself downward, keeping your arms close to your body until your head is about six inches from the floor.

- Push upward again, keeping your arms close to your body toward the starting position. Hold your stomach in tight to support your back. This completes one push-up.

- Do three sets of 10 to 12 reps, with a five-second rest between sets.

HIPS AND GLUTES

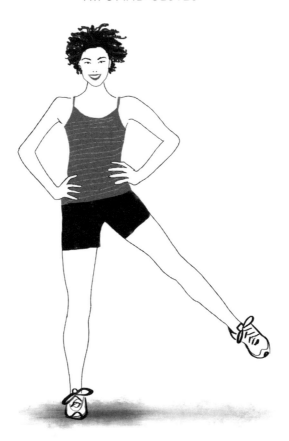

- Stand with your feet shoulder-width apart, with your legs slightly bent at the knees.

- In one motion, straighten your right leg while also straightening and lifting your left leg to the side. Use your quad and glute muscles to stabilize yourself, being careful not to lock your knees.

- Return to the starting position.

- Do three sets of 10 to 12 reps with a five-second rest between sets.

- Switch legs and follow the same steps.

- Variation: Add a resistance band or ankle weight for more hip and derriere toning. You will need a circular resistance band, or you can tie a knot in a straight band to make it circular. Place the band at your ankles while in the starting position. Be careful not to make the resistance band too tight or the ankle weight too heavy to protect against excess strain on your hip and knee joints.

STEP THREE: 10 MINUTES
CORE EXERCISES

Your core consists of the muscles that stabilize your spine and pelvis. They run the entire length of your torso and help keep you balanced as weight shifts when you move your body in different directions. The exercises described below are designed specifically to strengthen your core, though they benefit other areas as well.

CORE ROTATION

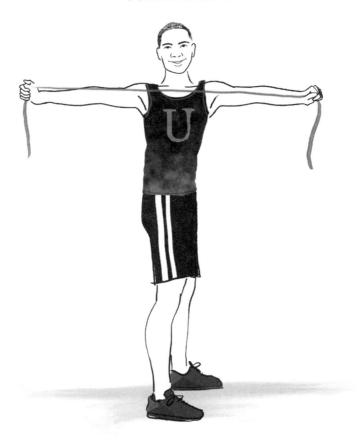

- Stand with your feet shoulder-width apart, your legs slightly bent at the knees, and your feet firmly planted. Hold your stomach in tight.

- Hold the two ends of a resistance band in each of your hands. Lift your arms straight in front of you at chest level. At the same time slowly open your arms apart to full extension, causing the band to become comfortably taut.

- Slowly and carefully twist your upper body to your right side while keeping the band taut and both arms in parallel alignment at chest level. Your right arm will follow the twist in your waist and end up somewhat behind you, while your left arm will follow the twist in your waist and end up somewhat to your side. Keep both arms in alignment at chest level and your feet and knees facing forward so that your twist comes from your waist and not from your knees. When you have twisted as far as is comfortable, return to the center starting position.

- Do three sets of 10 to 12 repetitions. Take little or no rest between reps.

- Rest for 30 seconds between sets.

- Switch the twist to your left side and follow the same steps.

To do this exercise with a partner, each of you holds one end of a resistance band in your hands and pulls it taut as you both twist in opposite directions.

- Do three sets of 10 to 12 repetitions. Take little or no rest between reps.

- Rest for 30 seconds between sets.

- Switch the twists to your other sides and follow the same steps.

FRONT STABILIZATION

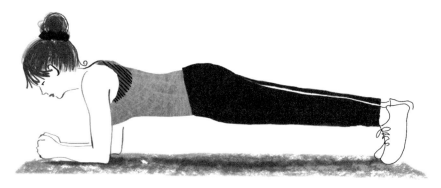

- Lie facedown on a mat or heavy towel in a standard push-up position. Slowly lift your upper body with your arms to reposition your elbows and forearms on the floor to prop you up. Slowly lift your lower body with your toes.Hold at about eight inches off the floor in sloping plank-like position with your stomach tight and back straight.

- Breathe deeply and slowly as you hold this position for 10 seconds. Increase the length of time as you get stronger.

- Lower yourself downward to the starting position.

- Do three sets of 10 to 12 repetitions. Take little or no rest between reps.

- Rest for 30 seconds between sets.

SQUATS

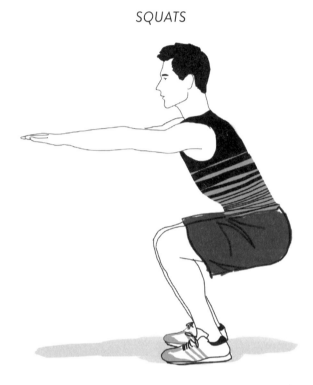

- Good posture is essential for squats so that you don't put too much pressure on your back, hips and knees. If you are a beginner, try standing with your back against the wall and your feet as far away from the wall as needed to allow for a 45-degree angle in your legs at the low point of the squat. Keep your body aligned to protect against excess strain on your back, hips and knees.

- Stand with your feet pointing forward hip-width apart squarely facing forward, and your head and shoulders squarely facing forward.

- Place your hands on your hips. Hold in your stomach. Slowly roll your pelvis backward so that your derriere follows.

- Slowly lower your body downward, keeping your weight on your heels and your knees bending no more than 90 degrees. Extend your arms straight out in front of you for balance. Maintain good posture.

- Lift yourself upward from your heels to the starting position.

- Do three sets of 10 to 12 repetitions. Take little or no rest between reps.

- Rest for 30 seconds between sets.

9

HEALTH TAPESTRY
WEIGHT LOSS PLAN: PART I

INSIGHTS AND MECHANISMS

As you age your metabolism slows down, and so does your hormone production. This life transition makes it harder to maintain muscle and keep off excess weight. More specifically, you start to lose the muscle fibers needed for strong, quick reflexes. In turn, the weaker your muscles, the more effort it takes to burn calories and stay toned.

High stress is another major factor in weight gain. When you are stressed out, your body often gets stuck in overdrive with your motors revving. As a result, metabolic changes associated with high stress get triggered—in particular, your cortisol levels shoot up. Then the dominoes start to fall one after the other: high cortisol causes fat to accumulate around your mid-section, as well as interfere with your good hormones that would otherwise help regulate your weight. The next domino to fall is often a feeling of exhaustion. Then another falls as your self-esteem suffers. And another as you reach for unhealthy comfort foods.

High stress also creates a catabolic effect, meaning your body breaks down more muscle than fat for energy, thereby causing more storage of fat. As body fat increases and muscle decreases, this makes it harder for you to keep weight off and increases the risk of many diseases. In both men and women, excess weight increases the risk of heart disease, diabetes, high blood pressure, high cholesterol, cancer, arthritis, osteoporosis and so many other conditions including acceleration of the aging process.

For women in midlife, hormonal shifts—especially in estrogen, progesterone and testosterone—can make that time period among the most difficult to maintain a healthy weight. Testosterone, which is present in both men and women, helps maintain muscle mass and bone mass. As is the case with high stress levels, the loss of muscle mass also results in a decrease in the burning of fat and consequently an increase in how much excess fat you store. Women who tend to store fat around their middle are sometimes described as apple-shaped, women who tend to store in their hips and derrières are sometimes described as pear-shaped. While "pears" may be frustrated by their heavy thighs, research shows they are at a lower risk for life-threatening diseases than are "apples."

For men, storing excess fat can force their testosterone to be converted into a form of estrogen that is possibly linked to prostate cancer, and the resulting lower levels of circulating testosterone usually leave them looking and feeling tired and flabby. One other stark reality for overweight men is that the more weight they gain from age twenty-five on, the shorter their expected life span.

But there is some hopeful news to come out of all of these findings. Numerous studies show that eating fewer calories may prolong your life. This sounds simple enough. There are some fancy terms we could use—systematic under-eating, calorie restriction (CR), low caloric diet (LCD)—but why bother? Simplifying in this instance is good.

So if you can remember only one guideline, let it be: eat less in total calories but not in volume of food. As we discussed for the Health Tapestry Weight Loss Plan, three to four pounds of food a day is the goal, but make them healthy lower calorie ones like vegetables. That way you will feel full as you're losing weight.

Let's put some more evidence behind this. The typical American adult is thought to be okay eating 2,000 calories a day. However, with a low-calorie diet, one between 1,500 to 1,800 a day, findings show life spans tend to be longer. This suggests that a lower caloric intake allows your body to modulate its metabolism which can then result in slowing the aging process. Fewer calories means fewer free radicals that damage your body. Free radicals are bad and the more you can do to stop them, like eating fewer calories, the better off you are.

By following our Health Tapestry Weight Loss Plan, you can take the guessing game out of how much and what to eat. For example, stay hydrated and half the battle is won; get enough sleep and you move even closer to your desired weight because thirst and fatigue often mask themselves as a hunger. Everything affects everything else. As you begin to implement the Plan, over time you will build some reserves for when a piece occasionally falls short, like when you have a sleepless night, and your body will self-correct without much trouble. But in the beginning months of your Health Tapestry Plan, be as diligent as possible. Because if you're like most people, not only are you lacking reserves, you are also paying a high price every time you have to borrow from one place to pay another.

Though excess weight is unhealthy no matter where your body stores it, having it around your middle is the most harmful kind. This visceral fat is "deep" and affects the way your body functions. It aggravates inflammation, alters hormone balances and raises the risk for high blood pressure, diabetes, early onset of heart disease and certain types of cancers. While the average woman may have 40 to 50 pounds of fat distributed throughout her body, somewhere between 5 to 10 pounds of it is usually concentrated in this deep fat. This is not the same as the belly fat you can jiggle and make jokes about. It's intra-abdominal so you can't see it or feel it.

Here is one example of how this deep fat hurts you. Trans fats and saturated fats found in processed foods, dairy, red meats and other products desensitize your body to insulin. This can lead to insulin resistance. What this means is the sugar stays in your bloodstream instead of being pushed out into your tissues where it is needed, resulting in high insulin levels. This is a big problem and the root of many diseases. Insulin resistance is often a precursor to Type 2 diabetes.

Your insulin levels are directly related to how much you weigh. If your body resists the effects of the natural process of releasing insulin into your bloodstream, then you tend to gain excess weight and keep it on. If your body goes along with the natural process, then you tend to lose excess weight and keep it off. The good news is that deep fat is the easiest kind to lose. In fact, if you lose about 10 percent of your overall body weight, that will amount to as much as a 30-percent loss of deep fat.

Interesting, you might be saying to yourself. *Deep fat seems like the place to zero in on first. But after I've done that, how much am I supposed to weigh?* There is no firm answer because so many different factors are at play, such as your body type, muscle mass, athleticism and self-image. However, there are two calculations we recommend as general guidelines. Neither is perfect so we recommend you use both.

The first is your waist to hip ratio (W-H-R) and the second is your body mass index (BMI).

To calculate your waist to hip ratio (W-H-R):

1. Take a measuring tape and wrap it around your waist at its narrowest point. Then measure your hips with the tape measure at the widest point.
2. Divide your waist measurement by your hip measurement. As an example, for a woman with a waist size of 33 and a hip size of 39.5, her W-H-R is 0.8; for a man with a waist of 39 and a hip size of 41, his W-H-R is 0.95. Current healthy weight guidelines recommend a waist-to-hip ratio of less than 0.85 for women and less than 0.9 for men.

To calculate your Body Mass Index (BMI), please visit any number of websites that offer free BMI calculators. For instance, the National Institutes of Health and the Centers for Disease Control are both excellent resources. Enter your weight and height into their calculators and presto. A BMI between 18.5 and 24.9 is considered best. If yours is between 25 and 29.9, you are considered to be overweight. A BMI over 30 is considered obese.

10

HEALTH TAPESTRY
WEIGHT LOSS PLAN: PART II

YOUR WEIGHT IS A RELATIONSHIP

If you follow our Health Tapestry Weight Loss Plan and implement our guidelines for sleep, physical activity and stress reduction, your weight will likely take care of itself. However, sometimes there is a hormonal issue, as discussed in the next chapter. Also, sometimes things don't fall into place as they should because there is a disruptive internal dialogue you have about yourself and your relationships with other people. These scripts, often playing on automatic mode, can be barriers to your health goals and well-being. Certainly being trim matters. But for some folks, it matters too much. Sometimes, rather than having a goal weight for your best health, weight becomes the lens through which you measure your self worth. The following patients' stories emphasize that sometimes you need to take a step back and listen to what you are saying to yourself.

Linda, a 46-year-old mother of two teenage boys, was depressed, mad at herself, and embarrassed about the 20 pounds she had put on since turning 40. Like a lot of people who get into a rut, she couldn't stop obsessing about the past. She reminisced about being at the peak of popularity back in high school when she had been a cheerleader, and as you might imagine, pretty, thin and happy. Guys asked her out and girls wanted to be like her. She was focused and made good grades. "It's not just that is was easy, it's that it all came so naturally. I thought everybody was this way, and if they weren't then they could be if they tried harder. I thought they must have been lazy, because if I could do it they could, too."

Now in midlife, she said to herself in the mirror, *what happened to me? I'm lazy, that's what happened.* Linda kept beating herself up, comparing herself now to how she remembered herself to have been in the past. She also compared herself to others in the present:

"I'm married—we argue, sometimes more than others—but we have two children together and the boys are everything to me. When they go away to college I don't know what I'm going to do. It's still a lot of work taking care of a family. I mean I love them all but I'm exhausted. But I see other people doing what I do and it seems like it's so easy for them, and they're not fat."

Linda had turned to food more and more often to comfort herself. It was easier than trying to drag her husband Charlie away from the Warriors, Patriots, Yankees, or whatever other urgency ESPN SportsCenter had to stop the world for.

At first it was a mostly healthy blueberry muffin from the grocery store. She really just needed to pick up almond milk, but felt like a treat too. Besides, blueberries are good for you. Then those chips Charlie likes, the ones with baked-in jalapeños and cheese, were on sale that week so she picked up a few bags.

A week later the "party size" of corn chips was on sale for the same price as the regular size. *Ten ounces more for free! We've got to have guacamole then. Anyway, it's fun. I'll watch SportsCenter with him. I'll ask him about LeBron James. We'll talk about Tiger Woods.*

But what started as an occasional treat became a habit. A night just wasn't complete without snacks. And the boys might even hang around for a few minutes to talk if there was ice cream. "Yeah, there's a reason they call it comfort food," she'd said to Charlie as they settled in for the night—after sports he'd stay and watch HBO with her.

Linda's nighttime treats carried into morning ones. At Starbucks it was usually a Skinny Mocha—*because the Frappuccino Blended Creme would mean I've given up*, she told herself, *and there's no way I'm going to do that.*

In fact, she got all excited when she saw that the gym on the way home from work had lowered their prices. So she signed up with a promise from the gym's personal trainers that they would help her "set goals and systematically work toward achieving them." She lasted for not quite two months. The $19 continues to be automatically deducted from her checking account each month. Sometimes she thinks it's a waste of money to keep it, but she likes having it as an option just in case she ever wants to go in for a quick workout and sauna. She hasn't been in six months, but said she's planning on starting back soon.

We have heard stories like Linda's from so many of our patients. In almost every case, they have one telltale sign in common: being overweight and the food choices they make are a reflection of their relationship with themselves and with others. Also, their breaking points weren't what they expected them to be.

For example, it turns out that embarrassment is what really started to make the walls feel like they were closing in on Linda. She was no high school cheerleader anymore, but she still wanted to look good. Wearing her hair longer and adding more blonde highlights helped give the appearance of being slimmer—at least that's what a fashion magazine advised in "10 Hairstyles That Make You Look 10 Pounds Thinner." But underneath the illusion she was embarrassed by her looks. It got to the point where she even refused to undress in front of her husband.

Charlie had also been a patient of ours in the past for a condition that was resolved. He's actually the one who asked us for advice during one of his medical visits because he was upset about the state of his marriage. "My wife is very pretty, and okay, she's put on a few pounds, but I'm still attracted to her. But we just seem to be growing further and further apart."

As you might guess, he'd also put on extra weight. For many couples, one or both of them being overweight can be such an emotionally charged issue that it's difficult for them to talk about it. That's why many of our patients find coming in to talk to us helps them address their challenges more constructively than by rehashing the same concerns and hitting the same walls.

Sometimes these couples meet with one of our mind-body therapists who helps them find their way back to happiness. One basic approach is an exercise with each person listening to the other without interrupting. Sometimes a constructive conversation that clears the air is enough to re-establish the commitment and intimacy that had previously nurtured the relationship.

For Linda and Charlie, living their separate lives had gone on long enough, and counting on the kids to be their middle ground wasn't going to work anymore. They had never wanted to split up, yet more distance seemed to be the only answer they could find. What had started out as giving each other space to buffer the intense feelings they were both experiencing had turned into both feeling lonely, with more loneliness on the horizon. To their credit, they both realized this at about the same time and sought our help. This first step allowed a bridge to emerge through the fog. "We can work this out," they started saying.

Through the Neuro Emotional Technique (NET), both of them quickly realized that their slump was about more than just their relationship. Linda gradually learned to reconnect with all that she had to be proud of once she worked through some of her past difficulties. NET helped her release her self-deprecating inner script and become more assertive about what she wanted in life.

Charlie had his own challenges. For example, he had self-imposed scales by which he measured himself. His mental scale measured finances. *If I had more money, I would be more of a man.* His bathroom scale showed him that he'd gained weight. He had been eating poorly to comfort himself on what seemed like a never-ending climb up a mountain of inadequacy. NET helped him to quickly realize that this thinking had started long ago. Growing up, nothing he did was ever enough for his father. If he won a baseball game, his dad would still find flaws in his pitching. If he came home with a 99 on a test, there was no celebration, just questions about why he didn't get 100. While the script of inadequacy may have pushed him to achieve, his unrelenting internal dialogue was killing him.

We knew a big milestone had been reached in their journey when the two showed up one day for a visit and Linda opened with, "Charlie and I decided to make a commitment to put our health and the health of our boys first. We're not taking it for granted anymore." We are happy to tell you that they have lived up to their commitment and both are doing well. They even took our mindfulness-based program and made it a habit to practice "mindful eating."

Their older son just started his freshman year at college. The other has two years left of high school. They're good with their parent's new awareness. The younger one asked his mom not to bring home fried chicken anymore. "Roasted is better for you," is what Linda told us he said. At first she was surprised because their family had loved the crispy, spicy, takeout. But after thinking about it, she realized just how much it meant to her kids that she and Charlie were taking better care of themselves. The very thing that she thought was not a priority while tending to her family's needs turned out to be the one priority they had for her all along. Self-care, instead of self-neglect, even if intended to be for the sake of her family, was the best way to give more to the people she loved.

Linda and Charlie also started having more sit-down meals at home without ordering in or microwaving something quick. They implemented parts of the Health Tapestry Weight Loss Plan into their routines and committed to strictly following the meal plan one week per month. They partnered up to get in some exercise. Snacking on chips gave way to snacking on brown rice crackers. Chocolate nuggets gave way to our trail mix recipe. Sodas to smoothies.

As another example, one of our patients came to us in complete frustration about her husband.

It was obvious that underneath Valerie's blustering was fear. Fear that her husband could one day suffer from his bad eating habits and that she and their kids could lose him.

"Stan is more than 30 pounds overweight and I'm really worried about him. But he won't listen. Really it's just an argument waiting to happen whenever I start to talk to him about it. It's like he'll snap back: 'Just worry about yourself and leave me alone!'"

We advised Valerie that a more effective way than talking to him about making healthy food choices was to show him how to do it. For instance, offer him some of the strawberry smoothie she was going to make for herself. If he said yes, then her usual almond milk, rice protein, vanilla extract, blend of acai and goji powder and vitamin C wouldn't make a difference as long as it tasted good to him. If he said no, then she should move on; maybe next time he'd say yes. She could be more proactive in how she prepared their meals and what she bought at the grocery store. Since Stan was not amenable to actively engaging in our Health Tapestry method, our thought was to help Valerie by slowly changing the things that Stan was accustomed to eating. Air-popped popcorn replaced greasy chips, saturated fats in meals were largely replaced by healthier ones, and over time, Stan lost some pounds and his mood lightened a bit as a bonus.

So many of our patients are frustrated by the people they love not taking better care of themselves. The correlation between eating well and feeling supported while doing so is strong; so strong that we routinely include relationship building tools into weight-loss plans.

This integrative, holistic approach is needed now more than ever to help address our national epidemic. According to the CDC's latest findings, 71 percent of American adults are overweight, and of those, 38 percent are obese, which puts them at a greater risk for serious diseases. Obesity is the second-leading preventable cause of death after smoking. The CDC also reports, alarmingly, that approximately 33 percent of American children and adolescents ages two through nineteen are overweight and half of them are clinically obese.

You may know firsthand how difficult it is to lose weight now as an adult even though you might have been trim as a kid. But for those one out of three American children now facing weight problems, they do not have the advantage of at least being fit in childhood, which makes the chances of carrying excess body weight into their adulthood all that much greater.

This points to a cultural problem, one that is being passed from one generation to the next. In a sense, being overweight has become normalized. As this attitude of normalization gains steam, it is reasonable to think that the situation can get worse.

That is, unless each of us decides we've had enough. Concentrating on your own health can help motivate the people in your life who are closest to you to take care of themselves too. Call it leading by example. You probably already see this in your daily life. Once you start taking better care of yourself, lose weight and look years younger, people will start asking how you did it. When the people close to you ask you about it too, their curiosity can be an opportunity for you to partner up and help them move toward a healthier lifestyle. From there build on some of the common ground you already share:

Shop Together. If your loved one won't step foot in the store, then at least go over your grocery list together. Be willing to make compromises. If they want Lay's potato chips, suggest the oven-baked ones. If they put a 24-pack of Coca-Cola in the basket, suggest instead a 12-pack and 12 bottles of flavored sparkling water such as Coca-Cola's Dasani pomegranate blueberry or pear kiwi. If they want Honey Nut Cheerios, suggest the original Cheerios that you can top with fresh blueberries.

Change is difficult for everybody. So going slowly and giving your loved one a chance to adapt in small steps to a happy middle ground is a more sustainable approach. Over time, the old choices will be forgotten and the healthier new ones will be what their body comes to expect.

Cook Together. Preparing meals together is not only good for your waistline but for your relationship too. Even if your schedules allow for just a few nights a week or only on weekends, cooking together strengthens your bonds. It builds communication, teamwork, memories and traditions. In short, it makes you happier, and happier people have happier relationships. One other result is you will likely find yourselves looking out for one another more. For example:

"Honey, those sun-dried tomatoes are high in sodium. Don't use the whole package, that's too much."

"All right." Thinking to yourself, *I didn't know that.*

Go to Sleep Together a Tiny Bit Hungry. Across ancient civilizations to today, people have gone hungry. In our current industrialized Western society where obesity is an epidemic, one possible explanation is that our ancestral memories of those food shortages, and even starvation, have evolved as survival patterns where we fill ourselves up while the going is good, even if the chances of actually running out of food are extremely rare. Combine that with common sense that no one in their right mind would want anybody to go hungry, and you might find it counterintuitive that we advise some of our patients to do just that: go to sleep hungry.

With three out of every four Americans and one out of every three Europeans overweight or obese, going to bed hungry is not as bad as it sounds. To be clear, we are not saying you should be famished, but being a little bit hungry is okay. You need a negative calorie count to achieve weight loss. One way to do this is by having your lightest meal in the evening. Many diet plans even contend that when you eat is more important than what you eat. We believe both when and what we eat are important.

When you go to bed feeling slightly hungry, your body is saying: "I don't have enough calories to maintain my body weight." Here is where you have to make an important decision. By not eating, you will make your body burn stored fat. Conversely, by eating, you will either maintain your current fat or increase it.

Exercise Together. Work on ways to get in more physical activity together. Sometimes this may include encouraging each other to do your exercising individually. Please see Chapter 8 on exercise for more tips.

11

HEALTH TAPESTRY HORMONE BALANCING PLAN

One of our seventeen-year-old patients described himself as a "walking hormone" when he told us that he was obsessing about girls, worrying about his acne flare-ups, and hating his parents for telling him what to do. "I swear I'm going to move to Los Angeles when I graduate because none of the girls in my high school look anything like models and I hear they're everywhere in LA. That place is lit!"

One of our thirty-six-year-old patients described how for the first time she felt happy and solid in her marriage with two children; the second one a newborn just ten weeks old. "I was always all over the map. Jumpy and agitated. I'm not going to say out loud the 'B' word, but I was one. Now I'm the 'M' word. 'Mom' and wife. It's good. Really good. I feel like maybe this time, for real, the raging lunatic with PMS will quiet down."

One of our forty-nine-year-old patients described how she's always tired. "By the end of the day, after I get off work, I'm exhausted. I usually give the kids money to go pick up dinner for themselves. I know it's expensive, and I'm a single mom trying to save for their college, but I've got nothing left. So I just make a salad or scrambled eggs for myself, sometimes a bowl of cereal. They won't eat that though. As long as they stay out of trouble, and they say they do, and I think I believe them—like no drugs, and if my daughter gets a boyfriend she knows to be careful. She's 14—oh boy, now it all starts. But they're good kids. They mean the world to me. I'm just too tired to do anything more than try to keep my head above water."

One of our fifty-four-year-old patients described how embarrassed he was feeling. "Can you tell me about those pills I see advertised on TV? Really, doctor, has it come to that for me? I mean I'm no stud anymore, okay, I can accept that. But I'm not ready to be put out to pasture either. My wife says just hugging is fine. Really? Who says that? Who is that 'fine' with? Maybe when I'm ninety."

These are widely different people, yet they share at least one thing in common—the effects of hormonal changes on their lives. If any of these stories resonate with you, the good news is we have some integrative solutions. We start with blood tests and other assessments, and the plan that follows usually includes our proven lifestyle programs. If you are fortunate enough to get your hormones under control through these wellness strategies, then bravo—you don't need to consider doing much more. The midlife dip in hormones can be manageable for some but is a free fall for others. Don't worry if the latter describes you; there are several options.

We have a lot of success with bioidentical hormone replacement therapy (BHRT). This is an important topic to clarify because of all the confusion and misinformation out there about hormone treatments. Bioidentical hormones are sometimes referred to as "natural hormones" to distinguish them from the "synthetic" non-bioidentical hormones used in basic hormone replacement therapy (HRT). Bioidentical hormones are synthetic too in that they are synthesized in labs; however their formulas are structurally identical to hormones produced by human ovary, adrenal and testicular glands, whereas non-bioidentical hormones are structurally different.

This distinction between identical versus different structures is important. As you may already know, updated research reveals that certain types of HRT for women—specifically progestin, the artificial version of human progesterone—is linked to an increased risk for breast cancer and cardiovascular disease. This point is critical: studies indicate HRT that includes natural human estradiol and progesterone is safer, and the benefits can outweigh potential risks. Even so, it's understandable that many women are wary of all hormone therapy, not realizing there's a difference between the bioidentical and non-bioidentical treatments.

There are also many women who know the difference and decide there is enough evidence and support from the medical community that BHRT might be worth looking into further. We agree, and prescribe this therapy on a case-by-case basis with an eye out for any red flags. In particular, we do a thorough panel of tests and review the patient's medical history to determine her suitability and risk of contraindications. More on our evaluation process in a moment, but as you might imagine, sorting through all of the variables requires a close patient-physician relationship.

Testosterone replacement is controversial, too, but for other reasons. More than 800,000 American men are currently using testosterone replacement therapy to treat low testosterone levels—fewer women receive testosterone therapy. Nearly all prescriptions for testosterone are for a BHRT form, which many people think is better. Still, some physicians question whether testosterone replacement is safe, and a sizable minority doesn't believe that men in midlife need to replenish sinking testosterone levels at all. Our experience has been that the careful use of testosterone replacement in the right man or woman can have dramatic effects on their quality of life.

If you are thinking of taking hormones, we urge you to strongly consider BHRT. The treatment is widely available and commonly prescribed, though the go-ahead largely hinges on your medical history, overall health and personal goals. Despite many large-scale studies intent on settling the debate, there are still lingering questions about its efficacy. We believe the available information is enough on which to base an informed decision, especially since the more recent findings are more favorable toward the advanced BHRT estradiol and progesterone than the older HRT options.

What follows are integrative hormone rebalancing plans for women, as well as one for men. We urge you to read both sections as a way to better understand your partner, friend, or family member and then help them make their most informed healthcare decisions.

HORMONE REBALANCING FOR HER

My husband and I are both doing bioidentical hormone replacement. Before he started on testosterone, he was always tired. So after he had his hormone levels checked, we discovered his testosterone was very low for a man his age. He had a testosterone pellet implanted and had an immediate return of physical strength and things corrected themselves in the bedroom, too.

I'm nearing menopause and while I was having other blood work done, I had my hormone levels checked, too. We found that my estrogen levels were dropping so I decided to start bioidentical hormone replacement therapy. I take estrogen and testosterone now. It has been a blessing. I haven't gone through any of the terrible symptoms a lot of women my age go through. My feeling is, why go through it if I don't have to? And I'm hoping it keeps me feeling young.

—MARY, AGE 43

There are two schools of thought when it comes to hormone replacement therapy for women. One group favors using it solely for treating menopausal symptoms. They believe that if a woman has symptoms so severe and nothing else can help, then she is best taking replacement hormones in the lowest possible dosage for the shortest possible time. They often don't differentiate between using bioidentical hormones (BHRT) or non-bioidentical hormones (HRT) unless the patient expresses a preference.

The other group favors using hormone replacement therapy strategically to help keep women stronger and healthier as they approach their later decades. They believe that hormones should be taken at physiologic doses, meaning doses that will bring the patient back to their youthful levels, to prevent age-related damage, preserve bone health and maintain a high mental and physical level of functioning.

We fall somewhere in between these two groups. Typically we treat menopausal or near-menopausal women who have come to the Marcus Institute of Integrative Health specifically for our hormone rebalancing programs. These women are already convinced they want BHRT to reverse some of the unwanted changes from getting older that affect bone health, sleep, vitality and quality of life. This is a reflection of a larger shift in our society about how we view aging. Increasingly, people are making conscious choices to rejuvenate themselves more and enjoy vital bodies and minds in their golden years.

We also treat women who view our program as a short-term solution for coping with severe menopausal symptoms. They may have concerns about the potential long-term effects of hormone replacement therapy, but they are so unhappy with their hot flashes, insomnia and mood swings that they're willing to try short-term BHRT.

The third group of women who seek us out for BHRT are those who were previously on HRT, but discontinued it because of the negative reports described earlier. They find our program to be safer, they like that it is strongly monitored, and usually find it to be highly effective.

With that said, we cannot make a blanket statement that bioidentical hormone replacement therapy is 100 percent safe for all women, which is why we require each of our patients to be individually and thoroughly evaluated before, during, and after treatment. For example, before we would prescribe this treatment for you, we would first do a comprehensive evaluation to (1) make sure you are in good health (2) determine whether you are a good candidate and (3) formulate a plan specifically for you.

Step one is a detailed description of your medical history, family history, and your current lifestyle. This alone may give us enough information to start making medical decisions. For instance, if you are a younger postmenopausal woman, BRHT may actually help you live longer. According to a 2013 study from Yale University, hormone therapy "is associated with a decisive reduction in all-cause mortality." However, if you are already in treatment for breast cancer, your tumors are estrogen sensitive which means hormone therapy of any kind could stimulate their growth. Clearly, this therapy would not be advisable.

In other cases the picture is far from clear. For example, if you are rapidly losing bone mass, and your grandmother had breast cancer but your elderly mother and your fifty-seven year old sister have never shown any indications of it, further tests such as a baseline bone scan (DEXA scan) will help us weigh the risks of you receiving hormone therapy to preserve your bones, especially during the first five years of menopause when bone loss is greatest.

Other tests, including a complete blood panel and profiles of your thyroid, liver and kidneys, are routine. If you report typical menopausal symptoms, the following tests are also routine ones in which we check your levels of key hormones. The primary markers we look at include:

TSH: Your body is designed to naturally release the thyroid stimulating hormone (TSH) to keep the right amount of thyroid hormone in circulation. Thyroid deficiency is not uncommon among midlife women as a result of thyroid function slowing down with age. Low thyroid function can cause unwanted weight gain and other issues. When this is the case, we do additional testing to confirm the diagnosis and then decide on the next therapeutic steps.

TESTOSTERONE LEVEL: Even a minor dip in testosterone as a result of menopause can noticeably affect your desire, energy, mood and bone mass. There are primarily three testosterone measurements—total testosterone, free testosterone, and sex hormone binding globulin (SHBG). In both women and men, most testosterone is bound by SHBG and released into the bloodstream as needed. Only a very small amount, two percent, is in the form of free unbound testosterone and more readily available for use by your cells and tissues. But as you age, this amount of free testosterone decreases while the amount of the bound type increases. As a result, you may show normal total testosterone levels (bound + free) but actually be deficient in the more readily available free type.

PROGESTERONE LEVEL: Naturally occurring progesterone plays an important role in maintaining your healthy emotional and mental functioning. When levels of progesterone sink too low, you may experience sleep problems and difficulty concentrating. But the most common symptom is anxiety. If you are like a great many women who tell us they experience high levels of anxiety, this test will show if a drop in your progesterone level is behind what you are going through, which is commonly the case.

FSH: In your menstrual cycle, the follicle-stimulating hormone (FSH) tells your ovaries to produce estrogen. But as estrogen production begins to wane during perimenopause and menopause, your FSH levels rise in an attempt to rev up the waning estrogen production. In premenopausal women, results showing FSH levels under 20 milli-international units per milliliter (mlU/ML) are considered normal, and over 20 are considered evidence of diminished estrogen production.

ESTROGEN LEVEL, USUALLY MEASURED AS ESTRADIOL: There are three main forms of estrogen in your body: estradiol, estrone and estriol:

Estradiol is the most important female hormone. It regulates your menstrual cycle, sustains your bone density, and fuels your mood, libido, brain function, skin elasticity, and more. Lower estradiol production is what triggers most of the symptoms you associate with menopause: emotional swings, dryness, hot flashes, fatigue, insomnia, difficulty holding in urine when coughing and laughing. Not surprisingly, estradiol is the primary estrogen used in BHRT.

Estrone has been regarded as the most problematic of the estrogens because its typical rise after menopause can potentially create the most serious health risks.

Estriol has been regarded as the least problematic of the estrogens because it has the weakest estrogenic effects of the three. Yet it still serves an essential function in regulating menopausal symptoms and diminishing bone loss and urinary tract infections, along with other benefits. It is most commonly associated with pregnancy because that is when its levels are highest, though estriol remains active throughout your life. Post-menopausal women comprise the largest group with low levels of estriol.

ESTROGEN METABOLITES: These are infrequently assessed but they tell an important story. Estrogens that are naturally produced by your body, as well as estrogens introduced into your body by hormone replacement therapy, toxins you ingest in your diet, medications with estrogenic effects, plastics, pesticides, and more, are all processed into byproducts called metabolites. These metabolites have different properties and behaviors. Just as there are good and bad fats, and good and bad cholesterols, there are also good estrogens and bad estrogens. Generally, methyl estrogens are good and catechol estrogens are bad. The good kind has not been linked to the promotion of cancerous tumors while the bad kind has been linked to encouraging cancerous tumors' growth. Although research is ongoing, we conclude there is sufficient evidence to show that a healthy or unhealthy combination of your genetics, diet and lifestyle produce more good or more bad estrogens respectively. This means there are some proactive steps you can take now. That's where another test comes into focus. It is designed to screen for ratios between good and bad estrogen metabolites.

For example, if your good to bad ratio is unhealthy, there are still plenty of reasons for hope that you can improve it. Cruciferous vegetables such as broccoli, kale, Brussels sprouts and cabbage contain high amounts of nutrients that neutralize bad estrogen. Though we recommend everyone eat lots of vegetables, if you have an unfavorable good to bad estrogen metabolite ratio we strongly recommend you eat plenty of cruciferous vegetables.

We also recommend three additional supplements that have been shown to detoxify bad estrogens—calcium-D-glucarate, DIM (diindolylmethane) and resveratrol. We designed and tested the multi-nutrient supplement named Lucentia Peak for Her® that includes these three estrogens, and we saw notable effects on the good to bad ratio. We discuss these factors more in Chapter 4, Weaving in Wellness with Nutritional Supplements, subsection Hormone Balancers.

Although this estrogen metabolite ratio testing is not usually part of most physicians' screenings, it is a regular part of ours. We believe it will eventually become standard protocol for treating and preventing sex hormone–related conditions.

In addition, if you have a history of fibroid tumors or spotting or bleeding, we recommend an ultrasound examination of your uterine lining and ovaries. This quick and painless test is a good way to detect any problems. Like breast cancer, many reproductive system cancers are estrogen sensitive and hormone therapy of any kind can risk stimulating their growth. In our more than twenty years of prescribing and administering bioidentical hormone replacement therapy we have found uterine cancer in only two patients. Though the risk is thought to be quite small, we respect our patients' decisions about whether the risk of BHRT is reasonable for them. This respect for our patients is grounded in one particularly vital reality about medicine: there are no absolutes.

Your body could be swimming in bad estrogen and you still may not get cancer while another woman with lots of good estrogen and a healthy lifestyle does. We believe that as research continues to mine for answers here at the Marcus Institute, at our affiliates, and at other esteemed institutions, we will be better equipped to proactively guide our patients toward the best hormone balancing treatment plans. For now, we are guided by the best available data combined with the unique needs of our patients.

Whether you want short-term menopausal symptomatic relief or long-term youthful hormone levels to slow the aging process, find a doctor with an expertise in all forms of hormone replacement therapy who can tailor a plan for you.

Another big consideration is the method for introducing hormones into your system. Depending on how many hormones you take—estradiol, bi-est (estradiol and estriol combined), progesterone, testosterone, and others—you may need to use more than one delivery method. The choices are skin patches, creams and gels, implanted pellets, pills and vaginal suppositories.

The most popular of these are weekly patches that adhere to your hip or lower abdomen. The great thing about patches is they are easy to use and deliver a fairly consistent dosage.

Creams and gels are the second most popular. Usually you massage them into your chest, abdomen, or preferably where there is little or no body hair. Creams and gels are particularly good choices if you are looking for symptomatic relief in the short-term. However, in a long-term plan for an ongoing balance of your hormones, they may not be the best choice as they often are inconsistently absorbed by your body. Over time your skin can even develop what is referred to as "dermal fatigue syndrome" and temporarily stops absorbing enough of the cream or gel. If this happens, you will likely need to change areas where you have been applying it, or switch to a different method or formulation until your body is ready to start again where you left off.

Although skin patches and creams and gels are most popular, we have found through clinical and laboratory assessments that specially formulated BHRT pellets are the most effective method for giving stronger and more consistent levels of hormone replacements over a long period of time. A pellet is about the same size as a grain of rice and is implanted just underneath your skin on your upper buttock area. It takes ten minutes and can be done right there in the doctor's office. Your prescribing physician must have special certification to do this procedure. We regularly do the procedure in our office with great results.

Each pellet is individually formulated to gradually release the hormone replacement into your bloodstream based on your prescription. For example, prescriptions for one of our patients include estradiol and testosterone pellets. Once implanted, they are virtually worry-free for four to six months until new ones are needed.

Though pills are what you are likely used to ingesting, we do not recommend taking most hormones this way because of their higher risk for side effects. For example, your liver has to go through an extra process with the pill form, and this makes estrogen and testosterone less tolerable. There is an exception though: we recommend BHRT progesterone in pill form because it is absorbed better with fewer side effects when taken orally. To be clear, we generally do not recommend HRT progestins in any form, pill or otherwise. Even if the formula is identical to the hormone produced by the ovary, its structure is completely different.

Lastly, vaginal hormone-delivering suppositories and creams may be appropriate for some women, depending on symptoms and personal goals.

Your local pharmacy can fill an ordinary hormone-balancing prescription just like any other prescription. For example, patches such as Estraderm, Vivelle and Alora; and creams and gels such as Estrasorb, Estroge and Divigell. It is possible that your doctor might prescribe a special, individualized formula unique to your needs, as we often do. Those will need to be filled at a specialty pharmacy. Your neighborhood pharmacist also can show you any over-the-counter remedies your doctor recommends.

HORMONE REBALANCING FOR HIM

I can't tell you the impact that testosterone replacement has had on my life. It's been a huge leap in terms of stamina, overall well-being and feeling healthy. I feel now like I did in my late thirties and I'm not exaggerating. When I was in my thirties I had this strong passion to work hard, play hard, and do other things. But by my mid-forties I was tired all the time. Within a week of receiving the pellets for the first time—which for me was the four to six month dosage period—I felt like an entirely different person in terms of stamina. And a side benefit, which I'm never going to complain about, started new life in the bedroom.

—JOHN, AGE 48

If you are a middle-aged man battling fatigue, a lack of desire for intimacy, and difficulty keeping muscle tone no matter how much you work out, we already have a suspicion about what's going on before you even step foot in our office. The arrows are pointing toward a hormonal imbalance, just as a middle-aged woman often experiences with estrogen deficiency when facing menopause. Only in your case it is with testosterone deficiency as you face what is sometimes controversially referred to as *andropause*—the medical diagnosis often used is "hypogonadism."

When we meet with a new patient, we run a series of tests. We look primarily at the same three measurements in men that we look for in women—total testosterone, free testosterone, and sex hormone binding globulin (SHBG). Most testosterone is the bound type and released into your bloodstream as needed. Only a very small amount is in the form of free testosterone which is unbound and more readily available. But as you age, the bound amount increases and free amount decreases. So your tests may show you have normal total testosterone levels (bound + free) but with a deficient proportion of the more readily available free type.

If it turns out that you do have low levels of testosterone, you likely will also have some things in common with our other male patients experiencing the same deficiency: obesity, heart disease, diabetes, and sometimes other conditions. This means your "andropause" may indicate wider health issues, or if you're in good health, it may simply indicate an age-related decline.

A recent comprehensive study also suggests that low testosterone levels can shorten a man's life. Starting in the 1970s, researchers at the Department of Family and Preventive Medicine at the University of California, San Diego School of Medicine followed 800 men, ages 50 to 91, who were living in Rancho Bernardo, California. In the early 1980s, the researchers found that about one-third of these men had lower than normal blood testosterone levels for their age group. Over the next eighteen years, this group with lower testosterone had a 33 percent greater risk of death than the group with normal testosterone levels.

More specifically, the study showed that the men with lower testosterone levels were more likely to have higher levels of inflammatory cytokines—markers for inflammation—which are major contributing factors to, if not the cause of, most chronic diseases.

Low testosterone levels in midlife may also be a sign of accelerated aging. From there, many psychological consequences can arise such as depression, anxiety and isolation, which often interfere with the ability to function at work, at the gym, and in the bedroom. Though low testosterone levels in younger men are rare, if you are among them you will probably have many of the same issues as older men—bone loss, poor muscle mass, excess body fat, low mood and low desire.

In most cases though, you can expect to go through life with healthy levels of testosterone as your primary hormone, while also producing small amounts of estrogen, progesterone, dehydroepiandrosterone (DHEA), and other steroid hormones. Your testosterone peaks at about age seventeen, and remains near that level until about age thirty, when you gradually start to lose about one to two percent every year. Depending on how much you start out with, this natural process of a one to two percent annual loss can be minor. If your testosterone loss combines with an estrogen imbalance, the unfortunate result can be a belly that sticks out even if you are ordinarily thin. If you are overweight to begin with, this hormonal imbalance will exacerbate the problem, and that problem feeds other ones.

For example, if your fat cells contain a high amount of an enzyme called aromatase, it converts your precious midlife testosterone into estradiol and other estrogen metabolites that have been linked to prostate enlargement and prostate cancer. So the more fat cells you have, the higher the risk that your testosterone gets converted into different estrogens. And the more you age, the more likely you are to put on weight—on average about one to two pounds a year starting in your twenties up until about your sixties.

You don't have to be a mathematician to see that naturally losing about one to two percent of your testosterone every year, plus putting on one to two pounds a year, which causes an acceleration of more testosterone loss, is not going to give you a happy number. This is one more reason to take up a healthy lifestyle: it can help your natural decline in testosterone levels go smoothly down a slope and not off a cliff.

Recent studies also may help explain what appears to be a correlation between low testosterone levels and dementia in men. In particular, testosterone supplementation has been linked to improvements in spatial and verbal memory in men with Alzheimer's. There also seems to be a correlation between low testosterone and blood sugar disorders, hypertension and other cardio-metabolic conditions.

Combine these scientific breakthroughs, the increase in overall public health awareness, and the population of baby boomers now in their fifties and older and you can better understand why the number of American men seeking testosterone replacement therapy has increased more than threefold in the last twenty years. A study published in the *Journal of the American Medical Association-Internal Medicine* showed that many of these men do not even have low levels of testosterone. Instead, they believe it will increase their amorousness and energy levels.

Sure, we have patients coming to us for those reasons. Frankly, they probably leave our offices disappointed because we tell them, "If you have normal testosterone levels now, adding more is not going to do much for you." We also talk with them about how all of those heavily marketed over-the-counter testosterone-boosting supplements claiming to improve performance, athletic and otherwise, are mostly unproven and can be potentially dangerous. Quite simply, self-treating with testosterone or so-called testosterone enhancing products puts you at risk and may reduce your medical options for other concerns.

However, to the majority of our patients who come to see us about this issue we say, "If you have low levels of testosterone, we need to find out why and determine the best way of restoring them, whether it's with the Health Tapestry Weight Loss Plan and Exercise Plan combined with targeted nutritional supplements, or stress reduction, or some other approach."

If all our methods have been tried but your total testosterone, free testosterone, and sex hormone binding globulin (SHBG) levels remain low, the next step may be to discuss whether you are interested in BHRT. If you are, then we run more tests to see if you are a good candidate. These additional tests include a comprehensive chemistry profile to check your liver, kidney and thyroid functioning and a lipid profile to look for any underlying heart disease. Other diagnostics are exactly the same ones for women. For example, we request a bone density test (DEXA scan) to check your naturally occurring bone loss due to aging. Several more tests are not identical but similar, such as a routine check of your key hormone levels though with different primary markers more aligned with male biochemistry, including the following:

FSH and LH: In the case of primary hypogonadism, test results will show your testosterone levels are low and follicle-stimulating hormone (FSH) and luteinizing hormone (LH) levels are high. This is an indication that your testicles are not making enough testosterone, causing the surge in FSH and LH for which a rebalancing plan is the usual treatment. In a case of secondary hypogonadism, test results will reveal your pituitary gland itself does not produce enough FSH and LH. Thus, your testicles have no feedback guidance, causing a decline in free and total testosterone. In this scenario a further workup is needed to better understand the pituitary dysfunction.

ESTRADIOL LEVEL: High levels of estradiol—a primary form of estrogen—is a possible companion of testosterone deficiency. If your test results reveal abnormally high levels, you are at a greater risk of producing a different form of estrogen that is carcinogenic, as well as experiencing enlarged breasts (man boobs), poor muscle tone and fatigue.

TSH: Elevated levels of thyroid stimulating hormone (TSH) may indicate a thyroid dysfunction, which in turn can affect your testosterone levels and mute your desire, stamina and pleasure.

Other related tests specific to men include:

DHT: Dihydrotestosterone (DHT) is a natural hormone vital to the male body's physiology and biology. Its power over, and affinity for, androgen receptors are two to three times more potent than testosterone. Higher levels of DHT increase the risk for prostate concerns, male-pattern baldness, and other male-oriented conditions.

PSA: A test named prostate-specific antigen (PSA) is designed primarily to screen for prostate issues such as enlargement or cancer, and can also reveal infections and inflammation.

If everything checks out and you and your doctor decide it is wise to move forward, then the remaining decisions involve the best dosage of bioidentical testosterone replacement and the best method for introducing it into your body. Regarding dosages, prescriptions in generic amounts can be filled at your local pharmacy. Or your doctor may prescribe an individualized formulation for you that you can have filled at a specialty pharmacy.

The methods for introducing the hormone to your system are creams and gels, skin patches and implanted pellets. Testosterone pills are completely out of the picture because they have an unacceptably high risk of harmful side effects.

Testosterone cream or gel is a common form we prescribe; in fact it is the most common form prescribed in the US. It's easy and works well for many men. The most common dosage is 2.5 to 5.0 mg a day. Rub the cream or gel on your upper arm, chest, or stomach at around the same time each day to maintain a consistent inflow. Often, within just a few weeks, your testosterone levels will increase and you'll feel more like yourself again.

As with anything you put on your skin, there is the possibility of skin irritation. There is also a chance of "dermal fatigue syndrome," which means that your skin might temporarily stop absorbing adequate amounts of the testosterone. If this happens, you will likely need to change areas where you have been applying it, or switch to a different method or formulation until your body is ready to start again where you left off.

Another common method is an adhesive patch containing testosterone that you attach to your shoulder or torso. We prescribe patches that last for a day or for a week, depending on your needs. A common dosage is 2.5 to 5.0 mg a day. Patches are easy to use and deliver a fairly consistent level of hormones. However, the adhesive on the patch can cause skin irritation and some men find it a bother to change the patch daily or weekly as prescribed.

The third option, pellets, are possibly the most effective at restoring your hormones back to their normal levels in the shortest amount of time. Implanting a testosterone pellet that is about the size of a grain of rice just underneath the skin on your hip takes 10 minutes and can be done right there in your doctor's office. Your prescribing physician must have special certification to do this procedure. We do the procedure in our office using only a local anesthesia to numb a small area. Once implanted, they are virtually worry-free for four to six months until new ones are needed. Each pellet contains up to 200 mg of crystalline testosterone. Based on your treatment plan, three to six pellets can release a dosage of between 600 to 1,200 mg spread out over a number of months. This process of slowly releasing bioidentical testosterone is similar to the way your body releases its own naturally produced testosterone into your circulation.

12

WEAVING IN INTIMACY

Ever since Julie's new boss came on board, she's been losing sleep and gaining weight. Tired, cranky and unhappy with herself, being intimate with her husband was the last thing on her mind. But it seemed to her it was always first and foremost on his.

"We're newlyweds!" he'd argue.

"Three years isn't a newlywed!" she'd shoot back.

"But you're only 34!"

For that one she didn't have a quick comeback and instead went in the other room and slammed the door behind her. The tension between them had gotten so bad that they had come to dread spending time together.

About a year ago, Alex, a 51-year-old accountant, started staying up late watching TV while his wife, Kathy, had gone to bed hours earlier. He no longer initiated playfulness, and when she made the first move he most often responded with:

"I love you Kat, but I'm tired. Maybe this weekend."

"Seriously? You've been saying that. I hate this schedule you pushed on me. Wednesdays and Saturdays. Now you don't even do that. You're not spontaneous. But you're not a planner either. What are you? You flake!"

She became more cold and distant as time went on. Meanwhile, Alex had begun to fall asleep in front of the TV, some nights not even making it into bed at all. Nine months passed with no affection, or even a meaning-ful conversation. He knew it couldn't keep on like this. A bomb was going to go off.

Stories like these are typical of those we hear from the men and women we see at the Marcus Institute of Integrative Health. They come seeking our help because maybe at one time their intimacy sizzled, and for various reasons including medications, age, lack of confidence, stress, relationship difficulties—the list goes on—now it's fizzled.

Others come seeking our help because they've never been the type to sizzle. They confide in us, "I'm thinking there must be something wrong with me because my friends tell me their stories. It's almost embarrassing to listen to them. I mean, I didn't even know people did that kind of stuff. But yeah, they do, and a lot of it."

The media bombards us with a different version of how things "should" be regarding intimacy, and you can't really rely on what your friends say as fact, mostly because people are reluctant to tell the truth about their private activities. Even when individuals remain completely anonymous in controlled sexuality studies, they still tend to over-exaggerate or under-report. For example, in a 2015 *New York Times* feature by Seth Stephens-Davidowitz, a large survey reported that respondents claimed that in total they had used condoms 2.7 billion times during the prior year. Okay, except there was one problem. Only 600,000 condoms were sold during that time.

These wide variances between fact and fiction in sexuality studies also cast doubt on how often people have sexual encounters, how many partners they've had, and how satisfying those encounters have been. There's not even a reliable understanding of what "normal" is. A study published in 2017 in the *Archives of Sexual Behavior* reports that American couples average being intimate once a week. Yet a separate highly regarded study revealed 43 percent of American women and 31 percent of American men reported having low desire. So who do you believe?

We can help you answer that question. What seems to be true with these studies is that answers to intimate questions that are potentially embarrassing to the participants tend to get underreported. In the case with those reporting low desire, it is reasonable, then, to think that the actual percentages are higher. It is reasonable because of the research we know to be reliable. For example, 75 percent of American adults are considered overweight or obese according to the Centers for Disease Control. There is an unequivocal link between excess weight and intimate bodily functions. By deduction, many of these 75 percent likely have some degree of sexual difficulty, with a lack of desire being among them.

There is also an indisputable tie to stress. On one hand, some of our patients seek intimacy to relieve their stress. "Feel good" endorphins pulsing through their body help soothe their nerves. On the other hand, some of our patients are so stressed out that they don't want to be near anyone, and instead get "feel good" endorphins by being alone. Chronic excessive stress is in a category all its own. Not only can it disrupt hormone production; if you are in fight-or-flight mode, your body's natural defenses shut down nonessentials, like arousal, to focus all of its energy on survival. Please refer back to Chapter 1 named Weaving a Health Tapestry: Reclaim Your Body, Mind and Vitality for more discussion of, and strategies for, dealing with stress.

Another factor clouding the picture of what is "normal" is that people frequently turn to alcohol to put them in the mood. In reality, it's not so great for that. Sure, for some it relaxes inhibitions, at least at first. But do it too often and it can kill your mood and lead to performance issues.

It is also fairly well known that marijuana can stimulate arousal and relax inhibitions. According to the latest research, that is true for about half of users. However, what doesn't get talked about nearly as much is that for the other half, marijuana has the opposite effect and can impair arousal and increase inhibition. To be fair, the research at this time is inconclusive and there are different components of marijuana, such as cannabinoids and THC, that need to be better understood.

There is conclusive research that reveals that food can be a stand-in for intimacy. For example, many people who report a lack of desire, or that their partner has a lack of desire, self-medicate by overeating. Many people distract themselves from life's challenges, such as intimacy, finances, self-esteem, and most everything else, by eating their feelings.

Our intention is to encourage your intimacy as you and your partner determine what is right for the both of you. By that we mean there is no "normal." How amorous you and your partner are is unique to the two of you. For every study that says you "should" be intimate twice a week, there is another that says you two "should" be naturally in sync, which may amount to intimacy once a week or once a month. The issue isn't so much what it "should" be but what you would like it to be, and whether or not that is in line with your partner. If the two of you aren't on the same page, or if there is a lack of intimacy altogether, then further exploration of the issue is warranted.

Being in the mood involves numerous complex systems including the hormonal, cardiovascular, neurochemical and musculoskeletal systems, among others. We try to help our patients understand this intricacy through a broader integrative approach. Sometimes, self-reflection and realistic self-appraisal and appreciation of one's own unique self are both the prescription and the cure.

Take Steve and his wife, Lisa. At first they dismissed what they jokingly called "his flat tire" as just one of those things that happens to guys who work their tails off trying to make a living. But when it kept happening, they both knew something was wrong. Steve didn't want to talk about it. Frankly, who would? So he tried to fix it himself. *It's nothing. Besides, I've never had this problem before and I'm too young anyway—25 and still rockin'.*

Lisa went along with his positive attitude, mostly because she didn't want to upset him. And it was true, as he said, they started dating in college and had never had any problems before. But after three straight months of abstinence, positive attitude and all, she starting prying more, trying to understand what was going on. Steve wasn't having any of that. In his words, he wasn't "in the right frame of mind." Still, she kept trying.

The more she tried, the more he shut down, until by the seventh month into their dry spell the topic had become completely off limits. At least verbally, but neither had stopped thinking about it. It became like the proverbial elephant in the room—always there no matter how much they tried to ignore it. At the one-year mark, the elephant had taken over and finally pushed them to come see us.

That's right, Steve was only 25 years old. Surprised? That's understandable, because just by reading what's on the internet and watching TV it's easy to think this problem only affects older guys. Not true. In a 2013 study published in the *Journal of Sexual Medicine*, an estimated one in four male patients with a new onset of erectile dysfunction (ED)—diagnosed as a man's inability to have intercourse within a six-month period—are under the age of 40, and nearly half of those are diagnosed as having severe cases. Adding to the under-40's distress is a generally unsympathetic culture that expects young men not only to perform, but to do so at a moment's notice.

That is a lot of pressure. In fact, ED in younger men is almost always linked to psychological issues. In this age of casual encounters, or what is often referred to as a "hookup culture"—the world's largest dating website, Tinder, boasts 20 billion matches in just the past six years (yes, that's 20 with a "B" for billion and yes the world's total population is 7.7 billion)—psychic pain can rule.

One of the results is that many of these young men suffer in silence. Too embarrassed to talk to friends, too ashamed to talk to a partner or spouse, they instead pull back and isolate themselves. Some choose celibacy until they figure themselves out. Others go for highly charged encounters, relying on pills or injections to get the job done and then leave—*at least I didn't fail that time* is what they tell themselves, and confide in us. Most are mercilessly tough on themselves and hold on to the pain of lost opportunities and humiliation.

For older men experiencing ED, people are more sympathetic. A man nearing his fifties has come to accept, and even expect, these difficulties. Add in a lack of exercise, high blood pressure, high cholesterol, extra pounds, and whatever else he is dealing with medically, and at some point he will likely realize that he can't outrun Father Time. All he has to do is watch a late-night TV comedy monologue to understand he has become part of a fun-loving punchline and to not take this too seriously. He's probably happy just to have another shot at intimacy "when the moment is right" as the Cialis ads promise.

Clearly this is a deeply personal topic. We see firsthand how our patients struggle with asking for help. If you are in this same boat, first know that you are not alone. No matter how your body does or does not respond to intimacy, there are millions of others going through the same thing as you.

Second, the desire to feel intimately connected to someone special is universal, whether you have sexual difficulties or not. Casual encounters may be temporarily satisfying, but the closeness you develop from a sustaining, meaningful relationship is widely regarded as being superior, both physically and emotionally. There is no moral judgment here. This is what the research points to, especially in the long run. Individuals in stable, ongoing, intimate relationships live longer, are happier and experience a deeper sense of community, among other benefits.

Researchers at the Universitat Autònoma de Barcelona analyzed data on Americans between the ages of 20 and 64 in relation to their health and marital status. Married people were more likely to have preventive health screenings across all conditions including prostate cancer, breast cancer, high cholesterol, and more, than were single people. This rate increased over the length of the marriage and is what the researchers termed the "protective effect."

In another study conducted at Carnegie Mellon University in Pittsburgh, married individuals had measurably lower levels of the stress hormone cortisol than single individuals. And though everybody has high to low fluctuations in their cortisol levels during the day, married people returned to lower levels faster than did singles. Other studies show married individuals have higher incomes, more employment stability, and lower rates of emotional distress and addictive behaviors including smoking, drinking and illicit drug use.

There are some caveats though. Happy marriages are the ones that bring about the greatest quality of life benefits. Unhappy ones can have harmful effects. With an increasing number of people choosing to live together rather than to get married—the US Census Bureau reports 21 percent of American adults are currently cohabiting, while 50 percent of Americans are currently married, having steadily dropped from 72 percent in 1960—it is interesting to see a considerable amount of research showing cohabitators fare better in life than singles, but not as well as those who marry.

Of course millions of healthy singles, whether never-married, divorced, or widowed, have fulfilling lives, and being single can result in a healthy lifestyle. In fact, as views towards marriage have shifted dramatically, there are now more single than married adults in the United States. According to the Pew Research Center, in 1997, 47 percent of Generation X said a successful marriage was "one of the most important things" in life. While in 2012, Pew reported only 30 percent of Millennials said it was.

This brings us back to intimacy. Many of our long-married female patients report having the best sex of their lives while others confide that they have little interest but participate more as an expression of love for their husband, which in turn gives these wives some emotional satisfaction. On the other side, many of our long-married male patients want to give love to their wives, but often think that earning money and having a powerful career is the best way to do that.

Older men and women are more likely to be taking one or more prescription medications, such as beta blockers for high blood pressure or serotonin re-uptake inhibitors for depression. In a 2016 report from the CDC, 85 percent of Americans age 60 and older take prescription drugs daily. Common side effects include lowered desire and numbed responses to stimulation.

Our approach is to restore an individual's amorousness as a part of their overall sense of well-being, and if they are in a relationship, arrive at what makes sense for both of them in terms of physical intimacy. Our Health Tapestry Intimacy Enhancing Plan is twofold. First, we start with physiological and biological considerations. For instance, if you are a man with a groin injury from cycling long distances, we usually start with advising you to get a wider bicycle seat. If you are a woman with a recurring yeast infection, we usually start with advising you to wear looser fitting clothing. If you are dealing with chronic pain from a bad back or other ongoing condition, we usually advise starting with minimizing the weight you put on the sore body parts. If pain acts up some of the time, but you never know when, we usually advise having some quick fixes at the ready so you two can change things up a bit without much thought. Simple positional changes, for instance, can make all the difference in the world.

For some physical issues, our lifestyle approach might be great for many but not quite enough for others, and medication is then added to the plan. As an example, in addition to other therapies, we may prescribe Viagra or Cialis if you are a male experiencing ED, and prescribe an estrogen suppository if you are a female experiencing pain from dryness.

Next, we go further into psychological considerations, many of which we wrote about earlier. This aims to help you see your situation realistically: accept your limitations, validate your strengths, and gain perspective on your whole relationship. We encourage including your partner in your physical and emotional intimacy journey.

If you are a woman, feeling comfortable with your partner most likely ranks very high on your list. If you are a man, it is important to you too but likely to a lesser degree. Studies show men more often think of intimacy as being task-oriented while women more often think of it as romantic. There are a number of ways this can be translated in your relationship. For instance, if you two are in a disagreement, as a woman you might want to work through what's bothering you before showing interest. As a man, you might just want to turn off your brain and get the gratification.

We recently saw a couple, Pam and Bill, who were having problems despite describing themselves as being happily married. But whenever he wanted to be playful, she would shrug and say, "Oh please, I'm too tired." And when she would reluctantly agree, Bill knew she wasn't into it—he told us, "It's like she's thinking the whole time: 'Should I get that blouse at Nordstrom's or wait until it goes on sale? I don't really need more black but it's cute and I can wear it to work. But my arms look so bad. I better not. It's too sheer.'"

During our comprehensive consultation, we discovered that their problems began when Bill signed up their eight-year-old son for Pop Warner Football after the two of them had agreed they would not do that. "No way. Kids get concussions!" Pam had been adamant. But Bill went ahead anyway. She was furious and immediately withdrew their son from the league. Bill's talking to her about being "overprotective," as he had done so many times before, wasn't cutting it this time, and neither was just an apology.

He said he signed their son up because he simply wanted him to have fun with other kids. Bill had grown up mostly alone without friends or much family support, and his folks couldn't afford Little League, Pop Warner, or much of anything else. Yes, he admitted they had an agreement, but the thought of their son missing out on making friends was more risky than their only child getting banged up a little playing football.

Understanding each other better ended up strengthening their relationship and their intimacy returned. By the way, the swim team turned out to be loads more fun for their son than football.

Bill and Pam had a happy ending. We believe we can help with more happy outcomes for individuals and couples. The issue isn't as much about having effective treatments as it is about having patients willing to openly discuss their intimacy. That's really no surprise though. Studies show that both men and women are uncomfortable talking with their doctors about these concerns. For example, in a survey of 1,455 men ages 57 to 85 published in 2007 in the *New England Journal of Medicine*, only 38 percent said they had talked about this with their doctors. A study published in 2012 reported that only 40 percent of women had talked about this conversation with their OB-GYNs. Most of the studies cite that patients often feel too embarrassed to discuss these issues with their health care providers.

To be fair, it's a two-way street—many doctors are equally responsible for the communication gap. *The Journal of Sexual Medicine* published a study in 2013 that revealed that although medical school students are taught about reproduction, contraception and sexually transmitted diseases, they receive little, if any, training on discussing a patient's intimate activities.

The confluence of a patient's and their doctor's apparent embarrassment is quantified in a well-regarded 2005 study entitled *Global Study of Sexual Attitudes and Behaviors.* This international research program included 27,000 men and women from 40 countries. More than 13,000 admitted to having sexual difficulties, but only 2,500 of them went to their doctor about it. For the entire 27,000 who participated, fewer than 3,000 reported that their doctor had asked them about any intimacy concerns over the previous three years.

Slowly but surely these conversations are increasing as the importance of human sexuality becomes more integrated into a proactive approach toward wellness. We face this awkwardness every day when treating our own patients. The truth is, we work to balance our patients' privacy while living up to our responsibilities to provide quality healthcare; that care often depends on us asking and our patients candidly telling us what is going on. Knowing about the presenting symptoms helps us determine the underlying causes.

If you are a man, this can be especially challenging because not only is there an unfortunate insinuation about your masculinity, but now you have the added worry that there's a deeper problem. As we wrote earlier, for men there frequently is.

For example, Theresa finally was able to drag Chuck in to see us. Let's just say "their horse never left the stable." They had been married for twenty years, so he rationalized that his lack of interest was just a part of growing old together. After hearing him say that for the last few months, Theresa began to think *maybe Chuck is right. At this stage in our lives, maybe it's for younger people.*

More time passed. But what finally got her attention wasn't that "their horse hadn't left the stable" coming up on a year now, it was that his overall health seemed to be steadily going downhill. This usually energetic, upbeat man was so exhausted at the end of the day that when he came home he crashed on the sofa for the night. She would bring him his dinner on a folding tray so he could eat and watch TV. Weekends weren't much different. His five extra pounds turned to ten. Ten turned to fifteen, and that's when she decided she couldn't keep quiet any longer. So she and her daughter, who was worried too, knew they had to have a talk with him.

Chuck was a third-generation carpenter here in Philadelphia. Hard work and hard times were what he knew. He lived by three rules: don't complain, family first, and never quit. And if there was a fourth, it could have been: doctors are a last resort.

Theresa started, "Chucky, we want to talk."

"What about?"

"You're putting on weight."

"So I'll go easy on the cheesesteaks."

"Dad, seriously," his daughter Kerry pleaded.

"You're making something outa nothing."

"No, Chucky. I think you need to go get checked out."

"By who? You know a guy?"

"Yeah. I know a guy!"

"I don't need him. I'm fine."

"You're not fine. You come home and never leave that couch."

"I'm tired!"

"That's the point. You're always tired. Something's not right. You need to be looked at!"

"I've been getting in overtime. How am I gonna buy you things if I don't get in some overtime?"

"Chuck! Don't make me say it in front of Kerry."

"What? What's the big secret? We're family."

"You know what I'm talking about."

"No I don't. What are you . . . hey Kerry, you in on this?"

"She doesn't know. It's between a husband and a wife."

"Mom, you want me to leave? This is weird."

"Uh oh. Kerry, you see your mother?"

"Dad, come on."

"She gets that look. I know that look."

"This look, Chucky?" Theresa asks.

"Yeah. That's the one."

"Then you know you can't win."

"Yeah?"

"Yeah!"

It was a good thing she did win. We gave Chuck a complete physical examination, including a careful medical history, as well as laboratory tests to check his blood lipids, blood sugar levels, hormone levels and more.

You know the saying "you can't judge a book by its cover?" Well, ED is the same. For example, it is often an early symptom of heart disease. A 2018 study by the American Heart Association found that ED can serve as a warning sign years before cardiovascular disease develops.

What this means is despite jokes about "just take the little blue pill," it's more serious than that and is often the first step in a more comprehensive treatment plan that includes some combination of diet, exercise, lifestyle changes and medications to bring down bad cholesterol, triglycerides and high blood pressure. In some cases, there is also treatment for an enlarged prostate, anemia, diabetes, kidney disease, liver disease, neuropathy and other concerns.

Unfortunately, Chuck's test results showed he had metabolic syndrome, which is characterized by a cluster of conditions such as obesity, prediabetes, blocked arteries and poor circulation, to name a few. Fortunately though, metabolic syndrome can often be reversed before it gets worse. The trifecta is to lose weight and bring your BMI within the 20 to 25 percent range, exercise moderately for thirty minutes a day, and eat according to our Health Tapestry Weight Loss Plan. Medications and other therapies targeting specific concerns are also considered.

In Chuck's case, we prescribed all of the above. Within a few months, his energy and overall health were back on track. Couples counseling was also a part of their treatment plan—this is not unusual for many of the couples we see; it is more often than not that intimacy reignites only after the couple is ready to start talking candidly with each other again.

Another one of our patients, Nancy, was an attractive forty-three-year-old artist who had been divorced for ten years before moving in with her fiancé Robert, a man fourteen years younger than she. She came to us saying that she felt like a complete mess. She said her divorce had nearly killed her and now she was feeling desperate about marrying Robert. Her friends envied her:

"Every detail, Nance. Oh my god, he's twenty-nine. Come on . . . pleeaazze . . . My Harold is so boring. At least I can live vicariously through you," Marissa, her best friend since high school said.

"All right. You remember Joey from algebra class?"

"Joey, the one who dated that cheerleader?"

"Yeah."

"You never told me about him. You—"

"Wait, before you say anything, it was just one time."

"Wow. I'm shocked."

"Why would you be shocked? Hello—you and Mike Parrey."

"Yeah, but we dated for three months. Everybody knew."

"Anyway, Robert reminds me of Joey."

"In what way?"

"That's all I'm saying."

"That's not fair. Harold snores all night. He leaves his dirty socks on the floor no matter how many times I tell him to put them in the hamper. How hard can it be?"

It turned out Nancy was just stringing on her friend. What she told us was that she and Robert had been arguing a lot—specifically, "He wants physical intimacy at least somewhat regularly, and although I would really like to, my body and my brain are not on the same page. I've been having hot flashes at night which make the thought of sex uncomfortable, and I have more pain and dryness than ever before, which gives me a kind of anticipatory fear about sex being painful. He's been patient and we've tried other ways of being intimate, but I can't relax because I'm afraid no matter what we do it's going to be physically uncomfortable."

Nancy was nearing menopause, and her hormonal levels were changing. More than that, her whole body was going through changes. Her mood and anxiety levels were all over the place. We explained that what she was experiencing was quite common for women in midlife. After some tests we found that her estrogen levels were low. Our plan for Nancy included low dose bioidentical estrogen hormone replacement therapy to improve those levels along with some bioidentical progesterone.

We also explained that as a part of her aging process, it was natural for certain tissues to thin out and for some of her other bodily responses to slow down. She was comforted to know that she was not alone. Women of all ages, even in their twenties, come in with their own concerns. But in virtually all cases, these conditions are treatable.

Postscript: Nancy and Robert just celebrated their third wedding anniversary.

CASE STUDIES

Patient: Lydia, age 38

Concerns: Weight gain, irregularity

Diagnosis: Perimenopause

Treatment plan: Health Tapestry Meal Plan, Health Tapestry Weight Loss Plan, multi-nutrient supplement program

Physician: Dr. Anthony J. Bazzan

IN LYDIA'S OWN WORDS:

Looking back on my life, I may have always struggled with symptoms that nobody understood. In all of my childhood photos, my abdomen is distended. I had to take liquid iron as well, which then led to me having to take laxatives at five and six years old. Unfortunately, people didn't know I was born with celiac disease and my mom did what she could, not knowing what was causing all of this.

I was an awkwardly overweight kid and adolescent, mostly in my stomach and hips. I swear I was born with cellulite. I got my first period at twelve and started getting leaner after my first period. I always had hot flashes and hormonal breakouts that got worse and worse into my twenties and thirties, often tied to my diet. My weight fluctuated from eighty-three pounds at my lightest to two hundred pounds at my heaviest.

Once my celiac was triggered and full blown, I developed chronic diarrhea and gastrointestinal problems. If I drank alcohol or ate sugar, in particular, my weight would skyrocket. I now firmly believe that it was from hormonal imbalances and nutrient deficiencies due to my celiac disease. I was not diagnosed with celiac disease until my late twenties, which left me with a destroyed gastrointestinal system.

I was told not to eat gluten, but given no further guidance about how to manage my health. I remember my mom walking with me through Whole Foods up and down each aisle trying to figure out what I could and couldn't eat. I had hair recession, gum recession, and was skin and bones. As soon as I cut out gluten, I blew up like a balloon.

I tried everything to lose weight and get as healthy as possible. The no-carb diet, paleo, herbal HCG, thermogenics, all kinds of workouts. I would have success, then gain it all back once I stopped. I tried every supplement on the market, or at least I felt like it. I was trying my best to be healthy, obsessing about it, and frustrated with limited or fleeting results.

I felt as though I was crazy, that I would never be able to find a husband, and I hated myself, often avoiding social situations due to how I felt or because of my gut problems.

I started reading all of the Suzanne Somers books about hormones, weight, sugar and toxicity in our environment. I then turned to my boss, because I knew his wife was doing bioidentical hormone replacement. Not only was Dr. Bazzan on Suzanne Somers's list, my boss's wife recommended him.

I was referred to Dr. Bazzan when I was thirty-eight. My periods were non-existent and my body was drying up (eyes, lips, needed lube to have intercourse and enjoy it). I was having trouble falling asleep and I had not had solid poops literally in years–I am talking explosive liquid messes. Even as I began filling out Dr. Bazzan's questionnaire, I knew he was the right doctor for me. The comprehensive, full-body assessment was impressive to say the least. Not only was his staff kind and courteous, Dr. Bazzan *listened* to me. He spent over an hour talking to my husband and me, going over every question I asked, going over every test result. What he discovered and communicated to me, which no other doctor had ever communicated, was that at thirty-nine, I was deep into perimenopause. I was in a highly inflamed state inside my body, and my bacterial/fungal levels in my body were off the charts.

Within my first few months of treatment, I started the Health Tapestry Meal Plan, progesterone, and took Dr. Bazzan's recommended supplements. It was like I was de-aging. Three months later, I was close to my goal weight and feeling great.

Dr. Bazzan has been with me every step of the way, answering emails, helping me with supplements and adjusting my hormone levels. I have about ten more pounds to lose, twenty pounds down since I first started with him, and I am working with him to balance my hormone levels. My stools are normal for the first time in my life and my gut is continuing to heal.

Now that I know I have the safety net of Dr. Bazzan and the Marcus Institute, I am taking a deep breath and trying to take it all one step at a time. Every day I try to make decisions that are better for my health, and I now know what to do. I am about to begin their mindfulness-based program. This is how healthcare *should* be. I never before had a health care team like this, and for the first time I feel like I have control over my health, I understand what is happening inside my body, and I have a plan to manage and improve my health.

Patient: Artie, age 40

Concerns: Fatigue, intimacy

Diagnosis: Testosterone imbalance

Treatment plan: Bioidentical Hormone Replacement Therapy (BHRT)

Physician: Dr. Anthony J. Bazzan

IN ARTIE'S OWN WORDS:

When this started I was a forty-year-old man. I was married for almost nine years and we have two daughters together. I had no issues with sex and my wife was pleased with my performance. For some reason though, we could not get pregnant with a third child. My wife's doctor said that she was in great shape and should be able to get pregnant. How could it be an issue with me though?

It seemed like all of a sudden my energy levels crashed! I was tired all the time. I went to see my family doctor and he said that it's probably stress and I needed to exercise. I told him that on a recent shopping trip I felt like I was being pulled into the floor. He said, "That's different then." He immediately ordered a batch of bloodwork. When the results were in, there was nothing of note other than that my testosterone levels were below the lowest range.

I was referred to a urologist who examined me and then referred me to an endocrinologist. After some tests the endocrinologist informed me that I had hypogonadism and there was no cure for it. I would have to use a testosterone gel for the rest of my life. I was on a prescription testosterone gel for several months with some improvement in my energy level, but not nearly enough. Bloodwork proved that too. My body just would not absorb enough. I was then put on a different prescription gel, which did less for me than the first one.

My endocrinologist then put me on testosterone injections. I had to get injected about every two weeks. That was one bad rollercoaster ride. I had big swings in testosterone levels. I had huge emotional changes. I would go from calm and understanding to a raving angry man in literally seconds. It was so weird. I would feel my anger level rising and I would explode. I didn't even feel sorry about it afterward. This could not continue.

I saw another endocrinologist at a top institution. After more bloodwork and telling the doctor about what hadn't worked in the past, we decided to try short doses of a drug that was meant for fertility treatment. This was given to me off-label and I was on it for one year. Since nothing could be found as to why my gonads where not producing testosterone, it was thought that we could jump-start them again. I truly thought I was going to die in my sleep for the first three weeks on that medicine. I would wake up gasping for air. A gasp that I can only imagine would happen after being deprived of oxygen for many minutes. I slept almost sitting up, but this only made it slightly better. After three weeks I adjusted to the medicine and my testosterone levels were higher. They were not great, but at least I was slightly above the bottom of the blood level range.

After one year I stopped the medicine and my levels plunged again. My doctor discussed my situation with a colleague and it was determined that my symptoms were idiopathic, meaning that no one knows why this happened to me or what is wrong, and that they couldn't fix it.

My wife and I were disheartened to say the least. Gels didn't work for me, injections were horrible and the jump-start had failed. My wife searched the internet in desperation and came across testosterone pellets. She read that these bioidentical pellets would match what my body should be making and within two weeks I should feel much better.

Determined to help me overcome this, my wife found Dr. Anthony J. Bazzan as a top doc in the region. His office was almost two hours away, but we thought that was a small sacrifice if he could actually help. My wife and I met with him and immediately felt comfortable with his planned treatment for my condition.

Dr. Bazzan suggested starting with four pellets at 200 mg each. The procedure is beautiful in its simplicity. The area in the hip where the pellets are placed is numbed and the rest of the procedure takes about fifteen minutes.

You can see the procedure on YouTube and it looks scary, but you feel nothing. Also my wife was allowed to watch because she was curious. She was very pleased with the skill employed by Dr. Bazzan and his team at the Marcus Institute.

It took me about two weeks for the pellets to kick in, but when they did, I had my life back! I had energy and my mood was worlds better. I started looking forward to doing things and going places again. I have had no side effects from them.

I've been on those bioidentical pellets for over four years now, and I will be on them all of my life. However, I have a great life again and it's a small inconvenience to travel to the doctor for pellets every five months. I think I will be even better than I normally would have been as I age since my testosterone levels will be monitored and kept at appropriate levels.

Patient: Frank, age 46
Concerns: None. Participant in a full-day executive health program offered as a benefit by his company
Diagnosis: Hyperlipidemia, Vitamin D deficiency, early stage coronary artery disease, anxiety
Treatment plan: Health Tapestry Meal Plan, multi-nutrient supplement program, biofeedback
Physician: Dr. Daniel Monti

IN FRANK'S OWN WORDS:

I'm a chief product development officer for a biotech company, and my company contracts with the Marcus Institute for its Executive Health Program. Prior to my day at the Marcus Institute I saw myself as someone who was in good health. I felt fine and was always in high gear to get my never-ending yet exciting work done. Since I like what I do I didn't see my eighty-plus-hour workweeks as stressful. I wasn't big on seeing doctors but my company pays for the executive tier to have this full-day medical program designed by Dr. Monti. My CEO went through the program and talked it up quite a bit. All of my colleagues were going through it and I was beginning to feel like I better schedule my day so I wasn't the only guy out.

I have to admit I wasn't crazy about giving up nearly a day of precious time, not to mention the extensive history and labs I had to complete before the day even happened. The one thing that felt like a positive is that

I'm a big sports fan and saw from the Marcus Institute website that the Philadelphia Flyers use the program and many of the famous alumni hockey players I grew up admiring were endorsing the program. So I decided to just go with it.

I have to say that I found the process and outcome to be somewhat shocking and at the same time humbling. To start, my cholesterol was through the roof as were my triglycerides, and my vitamin D level was almost undetectable. The last time these labs were checked they were normal, but I can't even remember how many years back that was. Some other risk factors for cardiovascular disease were also found. And when the biofeedback psychologist assessed me it was clear that my body was feeling considerable tension that I wasn't aware of.

The good news is that my cardiac stress test and imaging showed that I hadn't yet developed significant coronary artery disease. Dr. Monti used the metaphor, "the bridge has been weathered by the storms but it's still standing strong…for the moment." He had my attention.

My company had used other clinics for executive physicals in the past, and this is where the story would have ended: "You have some abnormal tests, go see your doctor and good luck." These guys at the Marcus Institute were much more hands on and wanted to work with my primary care doc (who admittedly I hadn't seen in years). The cardiologist at the institute, along with Dr. Monti, put together an aggressive plan to see if I could reverse things without going on medication. They gave me three months.

When Dr. Monti was customizing my diet he wanted to know every detail of what I had been eating. I led with, "I eat a healthy diet." He smiled and asked me to go through it. Without thinking, I painted a rosier picture than reality. I'm not sure why I did that, but it didn't matter. He knew.

"What are you eating at night?" he asked.

"Usually nothing, I just crash on the couch while watching TV."

"Do you ever bring any food with you to the couch?"

"Sometimes, I guess."

"What's your favorite?"

"Ice cream I suppose."

"How much do you eat?"

It was at this point in the conversation that I realized I was hiding from him and myself that I eat ice cream just about every night before bed . . . the good stuff . . . and a full pint of it. The doctor pointed out how this in itself could be causing some of the abnormal labs. He put me on a diet I could handle. Since chocolate was the flavor I needed to have at night, he gave me a low-calorie nutritional shake that I put in the blender with ice to make it nice and thick. It worked. I did my best to do the other parts of his diet plan as well. It was less painful than I thought it would be and to my surprise I lost twenty-six pounds. The labs got better, too.

An important part of my success is Dr. Monti's insistence that I involve my wife in the process. I said to him, "She'll just love this. She nags me all the time." Dr. M said to let her gloat about being correct because her partnership to make this work was worth it. He was right. And instead of gloating she was almost tearful when I asked her to help me. She would make the shakes for me and helped think of ways to spice it up with natural flavorings. She made an appointment for herself with Dr. Monti and we are both integrative medicine converts.

Another important take-home from the day was the assessment with the biofeedback psychologist. Dr. Monti explained her findings in great detail and talked about how the unchecked tension/stress in my body was increasing inflammation in my system and adding to my risk of getting sick.

I'm a scientist by training and I knew this sounded correct. So I bought the home biofeedback device the psychologist recommended and my wife and I eventually took the mindfulness program together, which was a great experience for both of us. We even got a gym membership together and work with trainers once a week. I really did a full three-sixty, and I have to say my energy and focus have never been better. The time commitment for getting things on track seemed so overwhelming at first, but the payback in terms of my new level of efficiency and that healthy feeling I have can't even be measured.

Patient: Marjorie, age 64

Concerns: Chronic illness, seizures, social isolation

Diagnosis: Pesticide poisoning

Treatment plan: Health Tapestry Meal Plan, detoxification program, multinutrient supplement program, bioidentical hormone replacement therapy (BHRT)

Physician: Dr. Anthony J. Bazzan

IN MARJORIE'S OWN WORDS:

Bill and I, both widowed, married in 1992 and blended our families. We were happy, hopeful and healthy. Suddenly, in April 1994, my health changed.

I developed tremors and a movement disorder. Over the next five years my condition escalated to seizures. Despite seeking help from many doctors, I did not receive an accurate diagnosis until almost the new millennium.

Finally I was diagnosed with organophosphate pesticide poisoning. I found an environmental doctor who helped lead me in the right direction, but I was still very sick. I was unable to work or travel. I experienced social isolation due to multiple chemical sensitivities associated with this condition.

In 2002 I learned via the internet that Dr. Bazzan practiced functional medicine and had expertise in detoxification, which I desperately needed. During my first visit he asked me to what extent I was willing to implement recommended treatments and changes to my lifestyle. I pledged 80 to 90 percent. The challenge began!

Dr. Bazzan offered a nutritional education program, which I attended. Following a series of lab tests I began receiving custom IV treatments, glutathione IV pushes and B-complex injections. Then bioidentical hormone replacement therapy was introduced when osteoporosis was detected on a DEXA bone scan.

Over time I extended the Health Tapestry Meal Plan to also becoming gluten-free and vegan, and I really enjoy my new approach to eating. My health dramatically improved due to the program Dr. Bazzan prescribed. I feel well most of the time. I am no longer on oxygen. My seizures have been significantly reduced both in frequency and severity. Thanks to the hormone replacement therapy my DEXA scans showed remarkable improvement in my bone density.

Following my second husband's death, I moved to an active senior community. I became an active participant on campus. I teach mahjong, co-ordinate religious activities, and volunteer with Project Linus. I can again enjoy the company of longtime and new friends. I treasure my reclaimed health and social life. These are gifts offered to me thanks to my knowledgeable, skillful and dedicated physician and amazing team at the Marcus Institute.

Patient: Gerald, age 50
Concerns: Weight gain, fatigue
Diagnosis: Hormone imbalance compounded by excessive stress
Treatment plan: Health Tapestry Meal Plan, Health Tapestry Exercise Plan, multi-nutrient supplement program
Physician: Dr. Anthony J. Bazzan

IN GERALD'S OWN WORDS:

My initial experience with Dr. Bazzan began more than twenty years ago, while attending a functional medicine symposium in Seattle, Washington. Though I had heard of him and his remarkable work, I had not met him personally until he and few attendees at the seminar got together for dinner. Needless to say, I was thrilled to be among functional medicine practitioners.

As a compounding pharmacist and nutritionist attending many such symposiums, I've found that these intimate group gatherings are where the most important information surfaces. As fate would have it, I also found a new friend, colleague and physician. As I listened intently to every word, my attention focused on this kind and caring man as he talked about his journey through conventional medicine and his struggle dealing with the misconceptions about holistic caregiving.

I have a history of moderately high blood pressure, diabetes and heart disease. At about age fifty I had gained almost twenty pounds. I had five years of extreme stressors that wreaked havoc on my health. I was becoming more and more fatigued and sleepless. My high vitality and libido were diminishing. Essentially the joy, exuberance and drive were no longer there. I was struggling.

After Dr. Bazzan's assessment, within weeks of starting his nutritional plan I began to feel like myself again. The Health Tapestry Meal Plan and supplement recommendations have brought me back to my prime. My weight is stable. My BMI (body mass index) and muscle mass are very good and my waist is back to thirty to thirty-two inches, down from about thirty-seven. I work out three times weekly, work about forty hours weekly at my pharmacy, another twenty hours doing carpentry and yard work, and find time to get to my hobbies of golf, hiking, skiing and playing music. I have felt stronger than ever and my enthusiasm for life has returned, if not improved. Last year I attended my fiftieth high school reunion. I had numerous comments on my healthy, fit appearance.

This recovery journey was not easy and I could not have accomplished it without Dr. Bazzan's careful assessment, encouragement, spirituality and his firmness. I will be seventy on my next birthday. I feel a fit thirty-five.

Patient: Erin, age 16

Concerns: Looking bad on prom night

Diagnosis: Acne

Treatment plan: Health Tapestry Weight Loss Plan, multi-nutrient supplement program with an extra focus on probiotics

Physician: Dr. Anthony J. Bazzan

IN ERIN'S MOM'S OWN WORDS:

A week before senior prom, my sixteen-year-old veggie-hating daughter Erin was freaking out about her skin, specifically pimples and more pimples.

Right away she took Dr. Bazzan's recommendation to eat as many fruits and veggies as possible (and now refers to them as "sunshine" after her visit with Dr. Bazzan), and to add vitamin D to her diet along with specific pro-biotics in the hope for a natural solution to clearer, healthier skin.

She started about a week before senior prom and her face was really broken out with a huge cyst on her forehead that was really disturbing her. It all cleared up within five days of adding these two supplements to her mul-tivitamin along with the detoxification foods he told her to eat! She can't say enough about it and even made a little SnapChat "public service announcement" to her friends telling them to eat healthy and get enough vitamin D if they want the same results she had!

Patient: Megan, age 36

Concerns: Headaches, insomnia

Diagnosis: Stress, poor nutrition

Treatment plan: Health Tapestry Meal Plan, Mindfulness-based program, Neuro Emotional Technique, multi-nutrient supplement program

Physician: Dr. Daniel Monti

IN MEGAN'S OWN WORDS:

I was having headaches throughout the day and couldn't sleep at night. I knew a lot of the problem was stress, which wasn't a big deal to me until I started having all of these body problems. The stress nobody could see, but the bags under my eyes they could. So keeping my appearances up was the tipping point for me. If you looked at me you'd think I had it all. A good husband who is a good provider, kids doing well, and generally all of us in good physical health except for slightly high blood pressure which I was trying to get down with exercise.

So things were perfect. I guess at least until I couldn't focus at work from the nagging pain and couldn't get my eyes to stop being puffy—the dark circles in just the right light made me look like a zombie. I had heard about Dr. Monti, and the integrative medicine program he heads up here in Philadelphia made sense to me.

One of the first things we talked about was that despite appearing to have everything under control on the surface, I had completely stopped taking care of myself. I guess I thought I'd never wear down. No kidding, once upon a time, career during the week and friends on the weekends was no problem. I was on fire. Dr. Monti helped me understand that the fire had grown too hot. Granted, pushing myself got me to great heights, like graduating from Princeton and marrying a fellow Tiger right out of school. But I began to realize that I was still compulsively pushing myself and it was catching up with me.

The first thing Dr. Monti did was explain that inflammation was a real problem and where it originated, from what I was eating, not eating, and the internal and external stress I was dealing with. In addition, I wasn't taking care of my body like I once did and exercise had gone out the window a few years ago. My nutrition was clearly an issue and he spent time customizing the Health Tapestry Weight Loss Plan to fit my work and family schedules. He also suggested a few supplements such as an omega-3 fatty acid to help with inflammation and we tried some melatonin to help with sleep.

One of the first orders of business was to take the mindfulness-based program offered by the institute. Dr. Monti helped me realize that the more I was present and aware, the better I would be able to take care of myself. In fact, I soon began to realize that I wasn't paying any attention to my actual needs and instead was constantly bombarding myself with what the doctor called "should" statements.

Dr. Monti strongly suggested I have a few sessions of the Neuro Emotional Technique (NET), and this was truly life changing. I learned from this approach that I was not congruent with what I thought I wanted. For example, as much as I wanted to be a success, I had a script going on inside my head that was telling me I would always fail. I wasn't consciously aware of how powerful this script was until the NET treatments elucidated my unhelpful mantra, and more importantly pinpointed the time in my life when that kind of thinking began.

When I was in second grade, I developed appendicitis. I had surgery but there were several complications with infections and more procedures. I ended up missing the last few months of school and was held back to repeat the year. This was devastating to me. Up until then I was a top student. But something completely out of my control ended my road to success. Without even realizing it, from that moment forward I never trusted the successes I had and felt the need to keep achieving more because I thought the rug could be pulled out from under me at any moment. The beauty of NET is that I discovered my core issue by using my body, making the process so efficient.

Clearing up this issue had a dramatic impact on me and was clearly a turning point in my life. I'm now getting to a more balanced place and the headaches have gone from a crippling part of life to a very occasional occurrence. When I do get one, I immediately use the new intervention tools I've learned.

CONCLUSION

As the debate over access to healthcare in the US rages on, the shift from doctors as your caretakers to doctors as your partners is taking hold. It is hard to know if the debate is feeding this shift or if the shift is feeding the debate. It's probably going both ways.

The end result is that each of us now must take more responsibility for our well-being. No longer can we count on the next experimental drug or miracle treatment breakthrough to rescue us from our unhealthy habits. Not because there isn't hope—there is a lot of hope, and we're excited to see where new science and technology leads us—but because of two main reasons.

The first is: twenty-five years—that's how long it takes on average for a new medicine to be discovered, tested, approved and end up in your hand. Each at an average cost of $3 billion. Here's another number to chew on: 90 percent of these new medicines will never reach you because the testing and approval process proves them to be unsafe, ineffective, or both. Those are long odds to bet your life on.

The second is: prevention is the best cure for illness. The Centers for Disease Control and Prevention reports that "chronic diseases, such as heart disease, cancer and diabetes, are responsible for seven of every ten deaths among Americans each year and account for 75 percent of the nation's health spending." With preventive care, though, we could save over 100,000 lives a year, and one of those could be yours or someone you love.

As a practical matter, none of us can be naive about the state of our healthcare system. On average, the US spends twice as much per person on healthcare than other wealthy countries—the 2017 National Health Expenditure data calculates $10,244 per American each year—yet we have the highest disease burden resulting in the highest total number of years lost to disability and premature death compared to these same countries. It's not all bad. We lead the world in survival rates for many forms of cancer and in a number of postoperative recovery times.

You don't have to be a wonk to know that we're a competitive, talented nation and the current disparity between healthcare expenses and lagging results isn't going to last. Something is going to give, and like it or not, you as the patient are caught in the middle. We doctors, in our own way, are also caught in the middle, as are well-meaning pharmaceutical and insurance companies, and farmers and food producers. We are standing on the shoulders of giants who went before us so that we can enjoy the longest average life spans in history—in the year 1900 Americans lived an average of 50 years; today it is 84.

That increased life span also gives us the opportunity to better understand what happens in the aging process, and with that comes a new set of challenges that were unimaginable just a generation ago. The Holy Grail was once longevity. Now it is becoming more clear that this pursuit must also include improving the quality of life. A more profound multi-faceted approach is needed, one that integrates all aspects of well-being—the physical, emotional, intellectual, mindful, social, nutritional, spiritual, and more. We are at the start of an incredible convergence of awareness and technology poised to create a new definition of what it means to be truly healthy.

The Tapestry of Health Plan is the most effective solution available today. It is preventive yet curative. Resourceful yet priceless. Rooted yet futuristic. We are delighted that you have taken the first step to learn more about it, and wish you a lifetime of good health and inspiration.

INDEX

ACKNOWLEDGMENTS

This book is a result of numerous important partnerships with those who have helped propel a revolution in how we think about health. Incredible visionaries like Bernie Marcus and the Marcus Foundation have catapulted Integrative Medicine to a level we could not have imagined a decade ago. Forward thinking leadership at Thomas Jefferson University, including a highly innovative president, Dr. Stephen Klasko, and a medical school dean and provost, Dr. Mark Tykocinski, have dared to elevate Integrative Medicine to full department status alongside the other medical specialties.

There are countless other people to thank—the full list would be a book itself. However, we would be remiss in not underscoring the importance of the many hardworking professionals at the Marcus Institute of Integrative Health, including our leader partners, Drs. George Zabrecky and Andrew Newberg. We thank our tremendous scientific collaborators across the university, other philanthropic partners such as the Coors Foundation and the ONE Research Foundation, and pioneer partners in the field such as Dr. Sara Gottfried. We also are grateful to the family and friends who bolster us every day, and to the many mentors who have guided us along the years. In addition, having a publisher like Kenneth Kales of Kales Press, who really got us and our message, allowed us to collaboratively create the best version of this book possible.

Finally, and most importantly, this work is a testament to our powerful partnerships with our patients. Our deepest gratitude goes to the many people we've encountered who are looking for a solution and who have the intuition to know it lies beyond a simple pill or test. Our daily journey with them and with everyone committed to weaving a vibrant tapestry of health motivates us to learn more, explore more, and continuously push the boundaries of what's possible for health and wellness.